MOTOR SKILLS

Harper's Series on Scientific Perspectives of Physical Education, edited by Rainer Martens

MOTOR SKILLS

Richard A. Schmidt

The University of Michigan

Harper & Row, Publishers
New York   Evanston   San Francisco   London

Sponsoring Editor: Joe Ingram
Project Editor: Ralph Cato
Designer: Michel Craig
Production Supervisor: Stefania J. Taflinska

Motor Skills

Library of Congress Cataloging in Publication Data

Schmidt, Richard A.   1941–
Motor skills.

(Harper's series on scientific perspectives of physical education)
Bibliography: p.
1 Motor ability.   I. Title.
[DNLM: 1. Motor skills.   WE103 S353m]
BF295.S25   152.3   74-4531
ISBN 0-06-045784-8

for Gwen, who helped in so many ways

CONTENTS

SERIES PREFACE

As has occurred in several other fields, the knowledge explosion in physical education and its collateral sciences—the biological and behavioral sciences—warrants a different approach for conveying introductory material. Traditionally, a basic course has used a single text that superficially covers everything, but sacrifices depth. The alternative is a text that covers one area in depth, but ignores many essential topics. Neither approach is adequate. Physical education has become too diverse for any one individual to write about all areas with complete authority. The developments in the behavioral and biological areas of the field have been too rapid.

The Scientific Perspectives of Physical Education series essays to remedy the instructor's dilemma of choosing between breadth and depth. It is composed of five volumes, representing the fields of physiology, kinesiology, psychology, social psychology, and sociology. In that order, the series moves from a biological emphasis to a social emphasis. Each science is included because of its obvious relationship to the other fields, as well as for its growing body of knowledge, which is a function of the amount of scholarly activity occurring within it. And, of course, each field is included because of its relevance for the diversified physical education profession.

The Scientific Perspectives of Physical Education series, then, is a direct outgrowth of the scholarly activity occurring in physical education and collateral sciences. Physical educators are now realizing the importance of reaching the introductory, as well as upper level, students with high-quality, well-written, interesting material. Rather than material based on speculation and conjecture, information that highlights the continuing and exciting search for new knowledge is being sought. This series is our attempt to place such material in the hands of physical educators.

Each volume is written by an individual actively engaged in research in this field. The approach of the series has been to focus on the reciprocal relationship between physical activity or sport and the subject area. More explicitly, the influence of physiological, biomechanical, psychological, social psychological, and sociological variables on physical activity or sport are considered, as well as the influence of engaging in physical activity or sport on these same variables.

Although the material is written for the introductory student in physical education, it presumes that the student has a basic understanding of the various disciplines represented. Within each area we hope to convey what is known today, what is currently being studied, and what needs to be understood. Emphasis is placed on content rather than method. Although method dictates the quality of the content, the authors assume responsibility for discriminating between quality and lesser research. Documentation of material has been used sparingly, primarily for recent work, in order to retain readability.

By no means is the series to be considered definitive within each area or for the entire field. Much of our knowledge is incomplete; our understandings are limited. But it is necessary to remember that the acquisition of knowledge in each area is an ongoing process. Each author has attempted to tell it as it is, not as what he hopes or conjectures it to be.

The series offers some flexibility because each volume is self-

contained and may be used separately, or as a partial or complete set for a foundations course. Although written for the
introductory undergraduate student, dependent upon the student's background and the curriculum, the series may be useful
at more advanced levels.

Rainer Martens

PREFACE

I have often thought that automobile mechanics, physicians, and educators have more in common than generally meets the eye. For example, they are all concerned with remedying problems manifested by the objects or individuals with which they deal. Also, they all require extensive knowledge about the structure and function of those objects, with a great deal of the knowledge being produced by someone else. The teacher of physical education seems to be no exception.

It seems logical to me that individuals preparing to enter these (and similar) occupations should be educated in such a way that they understand as much as possible about the structure and functioning of the objects of their attention. Of course, this is not absolutely essential, because one *could* employ a methodological approach to their education that would stress the classification of the various problems likely to be encountered, the symptoms associated with each problem, and the most effective procedures to follow to relieve the problem. An important goal would be familiarization with the index of a

large manual (like a cookbook), with lists of symptoms, classifications of problems, and appropriate cures. Such an education
might produce graduates who could, within limits, operate
fairly well in the jobs for which they were trained.

The disadvantages of this system of professional training are
obvious. The graduates would not really understand the functioning of the objects with which they are dealing because of
the emphasis on methods of handling problems; thus they
would be limited by the information contained in the manual.
If the manual happened to be incomplete—because it had become out of date or because it failed to list some rare malady—
the professional would be at a loss to cure the problem. Also,
if the manual was not readily at hand to consult at every
turn, many problems would remain unsolved. Clearly, what
the graduate from such a program would lack is an understanding of the functioning of the objects with which he was
to deal, an understanding that can be applied to new situations
as they arise and to the more effective solution of problems that
have been attacked before.

Most would agree that one of the major functions of the
physical education teacher is to teach motor skills. Therefore, it
follows that he should understand as much as possible about the
way in which his students perform and learn skills. He should
know how the various structures relevant to motor performance
function and interact in order to gain insight into "what is
going on" as his students are learning new motor skills. Consistent with this point of view, this book is intended to serve
as an introduction to the understanding of human motor behavior, stressing the processes that are in operation during the
individual's general performance, rather than focusing on specific applications. The focus of this book will be on what has
been learned from research on motor behavior, emphasizing
methods of research and reasons for drawing certain conclusions, in the belief that such information provides a more complete understanding of motor skills for the teacher of physical
education.

This book is the product of a great deal of effort on the part
of a number of individuals. I wish to express my thanks to our
departmental secretarial staff—Mary Daum, Marie Lacey, and

Janet Larson—for their skill and patience in preparing the typed manuscript. A number of students at The University of Michigan read the early versions of the manuscript and provided helpful suggestions for improvement. They are Dwight Edwards, Gwen Gordon, Barbara Kirkendall, Susan Moxley, Diane Ross, and David Russell; I wish to express my appreciation for their time and effort. Extremely thoughtful and helpful comments were provided by fellow motor skills researchers Jack A. Adams and Ronald G. Marteniuk, and I wish to express my gratitude for the resulting improvements to the manuscript. Finally appreciation is extended to the authors and publishers who allowed me the free use of the materials appearing in numerous figures and tables.

Richard A. Schmidt

CHAPTER 1 | HISTORICAL PERSPECTIVE

The field of motor skills is, and always has been, tied strongly to psychology. It is therefore not surprising that the developments in motor skills have paralleled those in psychology quite closely. (Irion, 1966.) Early research in motor skills began in the early developmental years of psychology with studies of telegraphy (Bryan and Harter, 1899) and similar tasks; at the same time, psychology was moving from its earlier philosophical and introspective approach (such as self-reports of perceptions and feelings) toward a more systematic and scientific approach to understanding human behavior. Before this turning point, about 1900, motor responses had been studied mainly because they offered access to the "mind." Thus, the early work by Bryan and Harter and a thorough analysis of movements by Woodworth (1899) appeared to be among the first systematic attempts to answer some questions about skills for their own sake.

In spite of these early studies in motor skills (as we know it today), there was very little motor skills research over the next 30 years. There were exceptions, however. Some work was devoted to handwriting proficiency, some to the way that practice sessions could be best structured with respect to the amount of rest provided between bouts of practice, some to whether it is better to break down skills into component parts in order to learn them more efficiently, and some to the retention of motor skills. Although various aspects of motor skills were investigated, the quantity of research was small and the level of understanding of skills and their learning was poor. It is sad testimony that there was no work done by physical educators, even when the field had defined one of its major goals as providing instruction in motor skills.

During the 1930s there was a sharpening of interest and the development of various early theories of motor skills performance and learning. Areas of interest broadened. For example, individuals began to study skills from an industrial point of view, with an emphasis on the most efficient way of carrying mortar, shoveling coal, and so on, in so-called time-and-motion analyses. Physical education researchers began to apply scientific procedures to the study of motor skills; notable early researchers in this area were McCloy (1934), with studies of components of motor abilities (see Chapter 9), and Espenschade (1940), with studies of motor development, maturation, and motor skills in children.

THE EMERGENCE OF
MOTOR BEHAVIOR RESEARCH

By the 1940s motor behavior research had begun to grow extremely rapidly. The reasons for this tremendous growth are many, but one of the most important was World War II, which indirectly provided research support for those who would study problems in gunnery, vehicle control (e.g., submarines), and so forth. In addition, the armed forces employed a number of experimental psychologists interested in motor skills to run various skills laboratories, which were supported entirely by the Department of Defense.

Theoretical Developments

Another reason for the rapid growth in motor skills research was provided by some new theories of learning, most notably that of Hull (1943). During the late 1940s and early 1950s, a number of experimental psychologists were busy testing some of the predictions from Hull's theory, and a great deal of data were generated in this manner. Although Hull's theory was not a theory of motor learning exclusively, various psychologists tested its predictions using motor tasks because the performances were particularly sensitive to the fatiguelike states treated by the theory. Although Hull's theory eventually proved to be an inadequate explanation of motor learning, the data provided by these psychologists are present today and tell us a great deal about the way that practice sessions should be structured.

Skills in Industrial Settings

The increased emphasis on skills in industry was yet another reason for the growth in motor skills research. The new fields of ergonomics, human factors, industrial engineering, and engineering psychology sprang up because many systems that used human beings were becoming so complex that the tasks within them were very difficult for workers to perform. A great deal of research was concerned with the "feel" of aircraft controls, the design of aircraft cockpit instruments, the methods and organization of assembly-line tasks, and so on. All of this research expressed an increased interest on the part of industry to view each worker as more than another machine on the assembly line and to attempt to make work comfortable and efficient for him. Much of what we know about motor skills comes from these settings.

Skills in Physical Education

Increasingly, physical educators have felt that an understanding of motor skills and their learning is needed for application in classroom situations. The father of motor skills research in physical education, Franklin Henry of Berkeley, made popular an approach stressing laboratory tasks, accurate measurement, and modern statistical analysis. Since his initial writings in the mid-1940s, he and his students have produced a great deal of motor skills work that is perhaps somewhat more applicable to teaching than is the work from experimental psychology. Since then, much of the physical education research has stressed tasks that involved the entire body and has involved questions relating to the structure of classroom situations, individual differences, motor abilities, and the like. The result of this emphasis is that today motor skills has become an important area in departments of physical education, and courses in "motor learning" have become popular in most curricula in physical education.

MOTOR SKILLS TODAY

It should be clear from the previous paragraphs that the body of knowledge in motor skills has come from a large number of fields and university departments and that only a small amount of what is known has come from physical education. The reasons that individuals have studied skills have been quite diverse, and that trend continues today. For example, there have been individuals interested in coordinated movements in nonhuman species, such as Wilson (1961), who studied wing-beats in locusts, and Taub and Berman (1968), who studied limb movements in monkeys. In addition, the emerging field of leisure activity has stimulated an interest in understanding the nature of play (e.g., Ellis, 1972), and there has been a growing interest in the area of rehabilitation that concerns the relearning of walking and other motor activities after injuries or illnesses.

As we have seen, the information that comes from physical education researchers for physical education teachers is only part of what is known about motor skills learning. Physical educators tend to dismiss the findings produced in experimental psychology or in animal laboratories because they "do not apply" to teaching situations. A more fruitful approach to the understanding of human movement is to examine all aspects of motor skills research from various sources to make conclusions about the basic nature of skills and their learning. As we pointed out earlier, with increased understanding the applications to physical education settings will be a great deal easier.

CHAPTER 2 | SCIENTIFIC METHODOLOGY

Exactly how science operates is a mystery to most undergraduate students, and this is too bad because the understanding of any area of investigation depends heavily upon knowing how the information was provided. This chapter deals with the nature of the development of knowledge in science; it does so without much reference to motor skills, concentrating instead on some rather abstract ideas. How these ideas apply to motor skills will become evident when various aspects of motor performance and learning are presented in later chapters.

THE STRUCTURE OF SCIENCE

Any area of scientific investigation is usually made up of four distinct elements, although very young sciences may lack one or more of these elements. They are observations (facts), laws, theories, and models.

Observations

Basic to any science are the observations about the things under investigation, which are sometimes called *facts* or *results*. These are directly observable outcomes of certain reproducible procedures; for example, "the population of Ann Arbor, Michigan, is 100,223 persons." Such a fact is tied only to the objects from which it was generated and does not apply to the number of dogs in Ann Arbor, or to the number of people in Chicago. Facts are not always easy to generate, as sometimes the procedures require expensive apparatus that itself might take years to develop.

Underlying the measurement of the population of Ann Arbor is the desire to estimate the position of Ann Arbor along the dimension that could be labeled "city size." This dimension is termed a *variable*, defined as *a set of mutually exclusive values that lie along some continuum*, and the value of the city size variable for Ann Arbor is 100,223 persons.

Relationships. Often one is interested in more complete information than the simple description of the value of some variable, and here one might be interested in the *relationships* among a number of variables; that is, knowing the value of one variable provides information about the value of a related variable. For example, knowing the value of the city size variable (100,223 persons) might enable us to estimate the value of the variable called "female population" at about 50,000 females. Variables can be related either *causally* or *noncausally*.

There are situations in which changing the value of one variable will *cause* changes in another variable. For example, increasing the variable "brake pedal pressure" causes the variable "vehicle speed" to decrease. The relationship is causal because brake pedal pressure was the only variable to change that was related to vehicle speed, and speed was not influenced by rolling down the window or turning on the radio. Notice that the *direction* of the relationship is critical: Changing the brake pedal pressure changed the vehicle speed, but slowing the vehicle by other means (e.g., hitting a tree) would not cause the brake pedal to "automatically" change its pressure.

Many relationships between variables are *noncausal*, however. Consider the relationship between the variables "shoe size" and "arithmetic skills"; in school children, those individuals with larger shoe sizes tend to have larger values on arithmetic skills. These variables are not related causally, however, because increasing the value of arithmetic skills (through a series of lessons) would not increase shoe size, and stretching one's feet will not increase the level of arithmetic skills. In this case, there is a third variable—"age"—that could be causing both variables to change. As age increases, shoe size increases through growth and arithmetic skills through experience. Therefore, age is a variable that causes changes in both shoe size and arithmetic skills, with the latter two variables being related noncausally.

In causal relationships, when one varies the value of one variable directly (e.g., by changing the pressure on the brake pedal), this variable is usually termed the *independent variable*, because its value can be set independently. In this situation vehicle speed is usually termed the *dependent variable*, because its value is *dependent upon* the value of the independent variable.

Types of Observations. An *experiment* is an operation designed to determine the extent and nature of causal relationships between two variables. In its most elementary form the experimenter sets up a situation in which he allows only one independent variable to vary and then measures the effect of this variation on some dependent variable.[1] Since an independent variable must vary in order to cause a related depend-

---

[1] Actually, some experiments allow more than one independent variable to vary in order to determine their effects on the dependent variable both separately and in combination, but such experimental designs are beyond the scope of this discussion.

ent variable to change, one holds all independent variables constant except the one under study; thus one can be certain that the changes (if any) in the dependent variable were not due to independent variables other than the one under study.[2]

Pseudo-experiments are procedures used in science that on the surface appear to be experiments but are actually not because they do not lead to the establishment of causal relationships. For example, if I divide elementary school children into two groups according to their shoe sizes and show that those "high" on the shoe size variable score higher in arithmetic than do those classified as "low," it would be incorrect to conclude that shoe size is *causally* related to arithmetic on this basis because shoe size was not the *only* independent variable allowed to vary. In addition to shoe size, we have such other independent variables as age and experience in school, which are systematically varying with shoe size. Although pseudo-experiments appear on the surface to be true experiments because many of the same procedures are used, they lack the one basic ingredient: They fail to hold all independent variables constant except the one under study; thus one cannot be sure which variable caused the observed changes in the dependent variable.

Interpreting Observations. As long as the experimenter has collected his data in an acceptable way so as to minimize errors, and as long as he has reported his findings truthfully, there is never any doubt about the "goodness" of those facts; the experimenter has reported his observations, and they are as they are. However, controversy may emerge in how those facts are interpreted. For example, if I find that Mary is 6 inches taller than John, that fact cannot be disputed; but if I interpret this fact to mean that girls are taller than boys, I would prob-

---

[2] Strictly, all independent variables cannot be held perfectly constant, but the systematic effects of such variables can be neglected by randomly distributing the variation throughout the experiment. For example, if the average age of two groups of subjects is approximately the same after randomly assigning subjects to groups, the systematic effects of age on the independent variable are said to be controlled.

ably receive a strong argument. Facts by themselves are not particularly interesting or informative, but the generalizations or interpretations one can make from them are; the next section deals with these generalizations, which are termed *laws*.

Laws

When a large number of separate facts or observations are collected concerning some class of objects, the general statements that describe these various findings are termed laws. There are many types of laws, but basically a law can be defined as *a statement of stable dependency between an independent and a dependent variable*. For example, I might observe that a spring elongates 2 inches under a weight of 5 lb, elongates 4 inches with a weight of 10 lb, and so on, each of these specific facts describing a separate set of measurements taken on the spring. With a large number of such observations, using different kinds and sizes of springs and weights, I might describe the relationship between the variables "amount of weight" and "amount of spring elongation" as follows: "Increasing the load on a spring causes it to elongate." Of course, a better expression of the law might be: "The elongation of a spring is proportional to the weight applied," this being the actual statement that has come to be known as Hooke's law of springs. Notice that the lawful statement applies to weights of any type, to springs of any type, and to the effect of weight on springs in all places in the world.

Such a statement has a great deal of power. First, it *summarizes* the results of a great number of individual facts in a single statement. Second, it allows one to "create new facts" without actually performing the measurements on specific weights and springs. For example, knowing that the law holds allows one to say that if a given spring is elongated 6 inches by a weight of 16 lb, it would be elongated 3 inches by a weight of 8 lb.

Laws, being the product of man's creativity in synthesizing existing facts, may be formulated differently by different people even when both individuals are examining precisely the same facts. If this is the case, how do we know which of the laws is the "correct" one? First, a correct law accounts for all of the facts; that is, assuming that the limitations stated in the law are not exceeded (e.g., a spring must be defined in a certain way), the law will predict the outcome of any test of spring elongation as it is affected by added weight. It is this principle that allows laws to be "tested." Once a law has been proposed, another scientist can test this law (1) by searching for existing facts that are contradicted by the law, or (2) by generating new facts to determine if they are as the law predicts them to be. Given that two statements of laws seem to satisfy the tests outlined above, then the "best" law is that one which is most simple (using simple mathematics rather than calculus), or most general in its application (applying to rubber, as well as to metal, springs).

Theories

The next most abstract element in a science is a theory, sometimes termed a *hypothesis*. A theory relates a series of laws to one another by means of an underlying *explanation* of the processes and mechanisms causing the relations between the independent and dependent variables. All theories consist of three distinct elements, although these elements are sometimes difficult to identify: hypothetical constructs, logical deductions, and coordinating definitions.

Hypothetical Constructs. Hypothetical constructs are the "building blocks" of any theory. They are imaginary entities with no formal definition as such and need not have any direct representation with some item known to exist in the real world. Good examples are Euclid's geometrical constructs, such as *point* and *line*. Although we have come to use the words point and line in familiar ways, Euclid's point and line were not intended to represent in any way the things that are normally called to mind by these terms. The only way that a hypothetical construct is "defined" is in terms of *postulates*, statements that indicate how the various hypothetical constructs relate to one another, such as "two points determine a line," or "two straight lines can intersect in only one point."

Logical Deductions. Having established the hypothetical constructs and postulates, one is able to produce various statements (preliminary laws) that "govern" the behavior of the constructs. One can deduce all of the laws of Euclidean geometry (such statements as "the shortest distance from a point to a line is the perpendicular to the line through the point") from a few basic constructs and postulates. Often these deductions are termed *predictions*.

The predictions from a theory are worded as laws, and this fact is useful from two points of view. First, if a theory is "correct," it allows the generation of new laws and therefore new facts before they are actually found in the laboratory, avoiding the enormous task of collecting a large number of facts and generalizing from them. Second, predictions provide a way that theories can be tested. By generating a prediction (law) from the theory, one can then either search the literature for facts that contradict that law or conduct an experiment to determine if new facts will be in agreement with the law.

Coordinating Definitions. The coordinating definitions, sometimes termed *operational definitions*, express the elements of the theory in terms of observable objects. For example, the operational definitions of a "line" might be the mark that a pencil makes on the paper as it glides along a straight edge; that mark *is not* a line, but merely a "definition" of a line in observable terms. Similarly, "physical fitness" (a hypothetical construct) might be "operationalized" using the resting heart rate. But resting heart rate *is not* physical fitness; it simply estimates it. By operationalizing the constructs one has the means for specifying the kinds of observations (or facts) that should be collected to test the theory.

However, there are often a number of observations that could legitimately be estimates of a particular hypothetical construct. For example, both resting heart rate and the time required to run two miles have been used as measures of physical fitness. Therefore, there should be some agreement among the scientific community as to the most appropriate coordinating definition for a particular hypothetical construct.

Testing Theories. A theory can be "tested" initially by determining if it accounts for all of the laws that have been established about the class of objects under discussion. However, if the theory was carefully developed, the theorist usually will have constructed the theory so that it does account for all existing laws, and this step probably will not be particularly revealing. The next step is to generate a new prediction (law) from the theory and conduct an experiment to determine if this new law holds in the laboratory. If the prediction holds, the theory is said to be "supported." The term *supported* has a special meaning here, however: that the predictions from the theory held up in the laboratory, not that the theory is necessarily true. The explanation for this can be seen in the following logical example:

If A is true, B is also.		If the car is out of gas it will not run.
B is true.	*or*	The car will not run.
Therefore, A is true.		Therefore, the car is out of gas.

The reason that the conclusion does not necessarily follow from the first two sentences is that there may be many reasons why the car won't run, such as a malfunction in the electrical system or a stopped-up fuel line. Because data can be collected that are in keeping with (i.e., "support") the predictions of a given theory, there is no assurance that the theory is true, for a number of quite different theories could predict the same law and fact. Therefore, providing support for a theory is not always useful.

A more powerful method in the testing of theories is to attempt to show that they are incorrect. (Platt, 1964.) For example, if a theory is proposed and predictions are made and tested, with results being *contrary* to the predictions (i.e., the predicted law does not hold), then (provided that the test is repeatable) there is strong evidence against the theory.[3] An example of how this form of logic works follows:

If A is true, B is also.		If the car is running, it has gas.
B is false.	*or*	The car does not have gas.
Therefore, A is false.		Therefore, the car is not running.

---

[3] Of course, more than one experiment is usually needed to determine that a prediction from a theory does not hold. However, an accumulation of such experiments dealing with a number of separate predictions will lead to an abandonment of that particular theory.

Thus, by showing that the predictions *do not hold*, one is in a position to reject the theory.[4]

If there are two or more "competing" theories concerning a given phenomenon, the most efficient method of determining which of the theories is true is to attempt to *disprove* one of them. For example, we could list all of the predictions of each theory separately, then notice those instances where the predictions are different. Next, if we were to do an experiment to test these two predictions, both of them could not be correct at the same time, providing grounds for rejecting one of the theories. An experiment that supports one theory and rejects another is frequently called a "crucial experiment" and is one of the most desirable goals of the scientist. For these reasons, it is frequently said that "science proceeds by disproof"; that is, when all of the theories that are false have been shown to be so by having their predictions fail to hold in the laboratory, any theories that remain stand a good chance of providing the explanation of the phenomena under investigation.

A Word of Caution. If a theory predicts that some change should occur (e.g., some drug should decrease movement speed), and an experiment to test this prediction fails to show that such changes occurred, is one to conclude that the theory is incorrect? Not necessarily, because the experiment could have been too insensitive (because of sloppy measuring techniques, inaccurate equipment, etc.) to detect that a change has occurred. The question boils down to "If I have failed to observe an event, does it prove that the event did not occur?" and the answer is no. On the other hand, if the prediction from the theory is that the change *will not occur*, and my experiment shows that it *does occur* (and this finding is repeatable by others), I have stronger grounds for rejecting the theory. Having shown that *something occurred*, it cannot be argued that my experiment was too insensitive to detect the change; while it could be that the change I observe is not

---

[4] As Polya (1954) has said, "Nature may answer Yes or No, but it whispers one answer and thunders the other: its Yes is provisional, its No is definitive."

representative of the "true" situation, at least my experiment is not insensitive.

Models

The term *model* is often used interchangeably with *theory*, but the two concepts actually have two distinct meanings. (See Lachman, 1960.) A model is a man-made companion to a theory that serves to "bring the theory to life" by stating it in terms of well-known objects. For example, in the theory of atomic structure, a molecule (a hypothetical construct) is envisioned as being made up of a collection of little balls, some of which are packed together to form a nucleus (neutrons, protons, etc.), with others spinning around the nucleus in various orbits (electrons). In addition, there are mathematical models of learning and computer models of the human brain.

Models are not absolutely necessary for the theory but are quite useful for a number of reasons. First, they make the theory easier to understand by stating it in real-life terms. Second, they make it easier to make predictions from the theory through the use of everyday objects whose behavior is easily observed, which aids in theory testing. However, many theorists have resisted models because they provide a real-world representation of constructs that may or may not have anything to do with the real world; a classic case is theory in mathematics. Also, models can put blinders on the experimenter by suggesting predictions generated from the model but not necessarily from the theory itself. Models, involving as they do the process of "reasoning by analogy" (if two things are similar in some respects, they are also similar in other respects), suffer from the weakness of analogies. For example, while a human brain might operate like a computer in many respects, there are certainly ways in which it does not.

EMPIRICISM

Up to now, we have been discussing the testing of theories, but there is an alternative point of view, termed *empiricism* by Adams (1967) and others. "Empirical" means "depending on experience alone without regard to theory," and one can imagine a continuum, with end points labeled "theoretical" and "empirical," which describes the amount of reliance on theory and theory testing in research.

THEORETICAL — — — — — — — — — — **EMPIRICAL**

The empiricist (see Forscher, 1963) collects facts for their own sake without regard to the theories on which they bear, while the theorist collects facts *only because* they test some theory. Bear in mind that both individuals collect facts in exactly the same way; the fundamental distinction is *why* the facts are collected.

The empiricist argues that more facts are needed in order that they can become integrated into laws. While it is true that some additional facts are needed, the theoretical point of view argues that enough facts exist right now and that we should be generating laws and theories to account for them rather than generating more facts. However, a second argument is strong in favor of empiricism; B. F. Skinner, perhaps the most well-known psychologist today, feels that the theoretical method puts blinders on the scientist, so that all he sees in his laboratory are the facts that bear on some theory, with all other facts being ignored. He feels that many useful facts are discovered by accident, without a theory leading to the establishment of that fact. The principle, for example, of "intermittent reinforcement" (that rewarding an animal after only a portion of successful responses leads to faster learning than rewarding after every successful response) was discovered by accident; the apparatus that delivered the pellets of food to the animals malfunctioned during the night, and the scientists noticed the increased lever-pressing activity as a result. (Skinner, 1956.) The fact that important information can be obtained without theory is a strong argument for empiricism. However, the theoretical position would argue that such instances are quite rare and that most facts remain "empirical minutiae" forever. (Adams, 1967.)

The main disadvantage of the empirical point of view is that it is *inefficient* in explaining the phenomena under consideration. Imagine the number of observations that must be collected in order that, for example, the laws of learning be outlined; there are countless variables to study, tasks to be learned, and types of subjects to be tested. In the process, the libraries and data retrieval systems become crowded with a great number of separate observations. Clearly, a more efficient method is to attempt to gather together all of the facts presently at hand and to propose theories to account for them. Then, by conducting experiments *only* to test these theories, we save a great deal of space in the journals and libraries and arrive more quickly at the theories that explain the phenomena under consideration. The payoff is great. After outlining a theory that is correct, we can predict all of the various separate facts concerning different types of subjects, tasks, and variables, because we understand the processes underlying the performances. Operating theoretically is not easy, since it is far easier to do experiments "because no one has done this particular study before," but the rewards of operating theoretically would seem to outweigh the extra effort.

BASIC VERSUS APPLIED RESEARCH

There is, in addition to the empirical-theoretical dimension just discussed, a second way of classifying research; this dimension is termed *basic-applied*. *At the extreme,* basic research is conducted with total disregard for practical application. The basic research scientist studies his problem "because it interests him," not because it is important to the solution of some pressing problem in the real world. Although his research may not be immediately applicable, the basic researcher is usually confident that his research will someday be applicable. *At the other extreme,* the sole purpose for conducting applied research is that it be of use immediately. In an industrial setting, for example, a researcher might be concerned with a problem of production efficiency; he cannot afford to do research that is not immediately useful to him and his company. The examples given above are extreme in an attempt to define the ends of the continuum more clearly, and most research lies between these two end values.

The basic-applied and the empirical-theoretical dimensions are often confused, but they are quite distinct and should be separated. The empirical-theoretical dimension represents the extent to which *theories* are used in the definition of research problems, while the basic-applied dimension represents the extent to which the research was undertaken to solve some immediate and practical problem. This can be represented in the following diagram.

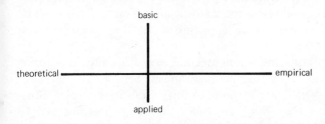

For example, an experiment in the upper right-hand corner of the diagram (basic and empirical) would have no immediate applicability and is not motivated by theory. On the contrary, an experiment in the lower left-hand corner (theoretical and applied) would involve testing a theory about something with great applicability (e.g., a theory of mental illness). While it might seem that applied research is to be preferred to basic, let's examine the question in more detail.

Applicability
The main advantage of applied research is obvious, namely, that it has immediate application to some real-world problem. It is therefore not surprising that applied research is so popular with members of the teaching profession, where questions concerning the classroom situation must be answered and applied as quickly as possible. Other less important advantages of applied research are that it can often be done with simple facilities, it is relatively inexpensive, and subjects are easily at hand.

Generalizability
With applied research there is often the problem of *generalizability* of the findings to other situations. If I conduct a study to determine whether method A or method B of teaching the

crawl stroke is superior, I will perhaps know a great deal about the specific effects of the two methods for the particular activity and type of subjects used, but what about the next practical problem that comes along (e.g., breast stroke)? I will not know very much about other situations unless I study them in the same way. Thus, applied research is inefficient in the long run. Imagine the great number of specific combinations of types of strokes, age and sex of the learners, and so on, that must all be studied before a complete picture of teaching swimming can emerge.

In contrast, one could operate very basically, the major goal being "to understand how human beings learn to move skillfully," with applications to any number of specific situations being some years off. Since this research is not tied to specific situations, as is the applied research, it has more generalizability to those situations, although the application will probably not be immediate. By knowing the laws and principles that govern learning and performance, we can predict the specific laws that apply to each new practical situation as it comes along, without having to run a new experiment for each new setting.

Experimental Control

A second problem with applied research is that of experimental control, and there are two major considerations here. First, doing research in basketball, for example, in an applied setting would require accurate simulation of the game situation, such as playing in an actual game with opponents, crowd, and so on. But such a situation is hardly appropriate for isolating how an independent variable (e.g., illumination) affects some dependent variable (shooting accuracy). By choosing a real-life environment, I have a host of uncontrolled independent variables and an experiment that is minimally sensitive to changes in the independent variable. It would be better, from an experimental control point of view, to ask that question in a laboratory situation in which lighting is varied for a task performed under closely standardized conditions.

Another problem is that many practical situations do not lend themselves well to measurement of performance (see

Chapter 3). Shooting accuracy in basketball, for example, can be assessed only by whether or not the ball went in the basket. Improved measurement can be achieved by using laboratory tasks that have a number of the same elements in common as the actual task but that have scoring systems more accurate and objective in nature. Laboratory tasks and procedures, while differing markedly from "realistic" situations, actually may provide *more* information about the actual situation than do applied studies because of increased experimental control.

Novelty

If I am interested in the effect of a new teaching method on the learning of motor tasks, and I choose basketball as my task, then I will likely have subjects who range from being varsity players to those never having seen a basketball. This results in great differences in performance among my subjects and decreases the precision of my experiment. The alternative is to use a task that no subject has ever practiced, ensuring a more similar beginning point for all subjects. Of course, this rules out most sports tasks and demands that laboratory tasks be used.

MOTOR SKILLS RESEARCH

The progress in motor skills research is somewhat retarded compared with other fields, in spite of the fact that there has been a great deal of motor behavior research conducted. Most of this work has been of the applied type, with one or more of the disadvantages listed above. As a result, the data are not particularly powerful in describing the basic mechanisms operating in motor behavior. What seems to be needed is a solid *basic* research effort, concentrating on the theoretical issues, in order to achieve the understanding that we need.

CHAPTER 3

THE MEASUREMENT OF MOTOR PERFORMANCE AND LEARNING

What has come to be accepted as "true" for motor skills is the product of research conducted in the field, and the application of the resulting laws and principles ultimately depends on understanding the research that produced them. In order to understand this research, we must know something of the methodology used. This chapter addresses itself to some of these methodological considerations.

CLASSIFYING HUMAN RESPONDING

Motor Versus Verbal Responses

One of the most useful schemes for classification of skills concerns the amount of "intellectual" involvement in the task. For example, a task in which the performer's major problem is "what to do" in response to a certain situation (e.g., press a certain button when a certain light comes on) involves learning which button goes with which light, and the main problem is conceptual; these tasks are often termed *cognitive, nonmotor,* or *verbal* and *involve a choice among well-learned responses.* By contrast, *motor* skills are those in which the subject's major problem is not what to do, but *how to do it.* The problem for the subject is *how to make a predetermined movement* more effectively (i.e., faster, smoother, with fewer errors, etc.). It is this second major classification of skills—"motor skills"—that is the major concern of this book.

This motor/verbal distinction is somewhat artificial, however, as all tasks have both verbal and motor components. For example, in an admittedly intellectual task such as a problem in mathematics, the individual must make a motor response (e.g., moving a pencil or the vocal musculature) in order to communicate the answer. Similarly, most tasks that we would all agree are motor (e.g., pitching a baseball) involve cognitive components such as deciding where and how fast to throw.

Classifying Motor Performances

Discrete versus Continuous Performances. If a task has a distinct beginning and end, it is usually termed *discrete*; a good example is a baseball throw and similar skills used in sports and physical education settings. A discrete skill may be either verbal or motor in nature according to what it requires of the individual, but a great many discrete "motor" tasks used in the psychological literature are heavily loaded with verbal components. A common example involves learning to flip certain switches when certain associated lights come on, where the problem is primarily what switch goes with what light.

When a motor skill has no distinct beginning or end, it is termed *continuous*, such as steering a car or running, which might continue for hours. A common type of continuous task is *tracking*, where the individual attempts to follow a target (e.g., a road) by making movements that control a *follower* (e.g., a car). There are two basic types of tracking tasks: (a) *pursuit tracking*, in which the subject has vision of the movements of both the target and of his follower (e.g., steering a car), and (b) *compensatory tracking*, in which only the error (the difference between the target and follower) is displayed (e.g., certain aircraft instruments). Because they are usually quite "motor" in nature, and because they are often found in everyday tasks such as driving a car, tracking tasks have been used extensively by motor skills researchers.

Serial responses can be thought of as discrete responses that have been strung together to form an apparently continuous performance. They have a number of distinct elements that must be produced one at a time in a particular prescribed order, such as starting a car, in which the sequential order of the movements of the various controls (e.g., ignition switch, clutch pedal, accelerator) is important. Serial tasks are usually, in the initial stages of learning at least, heavily loaded with verbal components; the learner can perform each of the steps easily by itself, but he must learn the proper order and time sequence of the various operations.

Open versus Closed Performances. A second method of classification concerns the extent to which the task is *predictable* to the individual as he is performing it. A task in which the environment is not changing and the performer can plan his movement well in advance without the fear of having the situation change is termed *closed* (e.g., bowling). A situation in which the environment is constantly changing is termed *open*; here the individual's major problem is to produce a response that can match the changing environmental situation (e.g., tennis, where the return depends on the opponent's serve).

SOME BASIC CONSIDERATIONS
IN MEASUREMENT

We now turn to some basic principles of measurement that apply to all branches of experimental science but that are especially important in measuring biological phenomena.

These aspects of the measurement process are (1) *objectivity*, (2) *reliability*, (3) *validity*, and (4) *novelty*, an aspect important specifically to motor skills research.

Objectivity

Objectivity implies that the performances are measured in such a way that any two trained observers or experimenters can arrive at nearly the same score for the same performance. Objectivity can be increased in motor skills by eliminating subjective evaluations by observers or judges, substituting the measures taken from various mechanical or electrical recording devices. The need for objectivity also limits the usefulness of many "everyday" activities for scientific investigation because most of them (e.g., dance) do not lend themselves well to objective measurement.

Reliability

Reliability concerns the extent to which a given measurement on the same subject under the same conditions can be repeated a second time. Errors in the measuring devices, such as irregularity in clocks or stretch in measuring tapes, contribute to unreliability but are generally small when high-quality apparatus is used appropriately. More important sources of unreliability are the variations within the performer caused by lapses in attention, changes in strategies, fatigue, boredom, and so on. These factors can be minimized by use of appropriate control over the environment in which the subject is to perform (e.g., tape-recorded instructions, noise-free rooms), but they can never be eliminated completely.

Validity

Validity is the extent to which a test measures what it was intended to measure. In order for motor tasks to be valid, they must first satisfy us that they are indeed motor (as opposed to verbal/cognitive) in nature. A second aspect of validity concerns the aspect of motor performance being measured, such as balance, speed, or steadiness. If the researcher is attempting to make a statement about the influence of some independent variable on balance, he must have a task that is a valid measure of this aspect of motor responding. On the other hand, the main question of investigations frequently concerns the effect of an independent variable on motor performance *generally*, and the task simply serves as a means of generating a score that is reliable, objective, and motor. In choosing a task that will most easily answer the basic research question at hand, many tasks are not clearly representative of anything for which we have a label such as *balance*.

Novelty

While not important to most sciences, novelty is important to motor skills because of the vast amount of past experience subjects bring with them into the laboratories. For example, if the concern is with the underlying motor abilities in human performance, we cannot test individuals who have had various amounts of practice with the task because we are never sure whether "good" scores are representative of a great deal of natural ability, a great deal of practice, or both. Also, in studying learning, choosing learning tasks on which all subjects have had extensive practice (e.g., throwing balls) or only some subjects have had extensive practice (e.g., playing hockey) presents obvious problems in studying improvement with practice. For this reason, many of the sports skills have to be eliminated for research consideration.

ASSESSING MOTOR PERFORMANCE

For most motor tasks, how well individuals perform can be estimated by some combination of three types of measurement: (1) accuracy, (2) speed, or (3) response magnitude.

Accuracy

One of the most useful methods for assessing performance is in terms of the amount of error the subject makes as he performs a task requiring accuracy. Accuracy can be required in a wide variety of ways, such as accuracy in reproducing a particular force, movement speed, or movement distance. An important aspect of performance in which accuracy is demanded is *tim-*

ing, where the individual must produce a given response at the proper time. To score accuracy, we can measure performance on a pass/fail basis, such as whether or not the subject completes a basketball free throw. At a more sophisticated level, we can assess the *amount* and nature of the error produced by obtaining estimates of (1) the average magnitude (i.e., direction, force, distance, etc.) via *constant error,* and the average inconsistency in producing the movements via either (2) *variable error* or (3) *absolute error.*

Constant error. Consider a task in which a blindfolded individual is to move a hand-operated slide a distance of exactly 12 inches from a fixed starting position. If, instead of moving 12 inches, he moved only 10 inches, he has made an error of 2 inches. If we let the correct response represent zero error, with short movements being negative and long responses positive, constant error would be -2 inches. If the individual were to complete 4 more responses with distances of 11, 14, 13, and 9 inches, respectively, he would have an *average* constant error of $((-2) + (-1) + (+2) + (+1) + (-3))/5 = -0.60$ inches. Notice that the signs of all the responses are taken into account when the scores are averaged and that the average constant error carries the sign as well. The meaning of this score is that the subject tended to respond, on the average, slightly (0.60 inches) short of the correct target. Constant error might not satisfy some as a measure of accuracy because the subject was never as close as 0.60 inches in any of his responses (the positive and negative constant errors "canceled each other out" when the scores were averaged). For this reason, either variable error or absolute error is also used because they are sensitive to the *inconsistency* of the subject in trying to achieve the correct target. Constant error is sometimes termed *algebraic error.*

Variable error. Variable error reflects the extent to which the subject tends to repeat his responses (or, conversely, the extent to which he is inconsistent) and is defined as the variability of the subject's performances about his *own* mean performance (i.e., his constant error). This variability is usually expressed as a standard deviation of the subject's scores computed over a number of separate observations,

$$\text{Variable Error} = \text{VE} = \sqrt{\dfrac{\sum\limits_{t=1}^{n} (X_t - CE)^2}{n}} \qquad (1)$$

where t is the trial number, n is the number of trials, X_t is the signed score for trial t, and CE is the subject's constant error for the group of trials in question. In the hypothetical example provided in the previous section, the subject's variable error would be

$$\text{VE} = \sqrt{\dfrac{(-2 - (-.60))^2 + (-1 - (-.60))^2 + \cdots + (-3 - (-.60))^2}{5}} \qquad (2)$$

$$\text{VE} = \sqrt{\dfrac{2.96 + 0.16 + 6.76 + 2.56 + 5.76}{5}}$$

$$= \sqrt{\dfrac{18.20}{5}} = 1.91 \text{ inches} \qquad (3)$$

Notice that the variable error is sensitive to the amount that the subject varies *within himself*. If every score were the same, each score would equal the constant error, and the numerator of equation 1 would be zero, with VE = 0 also; as the variability of the movements increases, the variable error increases as well.

Absolute error. While variable error is usually preferred as a measure of the inconsistency of the subject's responding, absolute error, which under most conditions is also sensitive to this inconsistency, has been widely used as a measure of error. The absolute error is literally the "average amount by which the subject was in error" and is computed as the average difference (ignoring the direction of the error) between the subject's responses and the correct response. In the example used above the average absolute error (AE) would be (where $|2|$ means the absolute value of -2, or 2)

$$AE = \frac{|\ 10 - 12\ | + |\ 11 - 12\ | + \cdots + |\ 9 - 12\ |}{5} \qquad (4)$$

$$AE = \frac{(2) + (1) + (2) + (1) + (3)}{5} = 1.80 \text{ inches} \qquad (5)$$

This measure indicates that on the average the responses were 1.8 inches off, but it tells us nothing about whether the responses tended to be long or short.

Recent evidence (Schutz and Roy, 1973) has pointed out that the constant error and variable error present clearly distinct and nonoverlapping information about accuracy in responding and that both of these scores are required to describe the subject's accuracy completely. Absolute error is a complex combination of constant error and variable error.

Response Speed

Response speed concerns how quickly the subject can accomplish a given task. One important classification is termed *reaction time* (RT), defined as the time from an unanticipated signal until the *beginning* of overt movement; for example, the subject is to lift his finger from a response key as quickly as possible after a light comes on. Movement speed, broadly defined, concerns how quickly a subject can complete a defined movement or series of movements. Another speed measurement concerns the number of acts that can be accomplished in a given amount of time, such as how many times a subject can tap his finger in 20 sec or how many telephones can be assembled in 1 hr by factory workers. A problem exists in using measures of speed, as many tasks that require speed also require some degree of accuracy. Generally, requiring greater speed leads to greater numbers of errors, this phenomenon being termed the *speed-accuracy trade-off*. It is a problem because how fast the subject can go will depend on how many errors he is allowed or is willing to make. Such tasks with conflicting goals (speed versus accuracy) are difficult to deal with in motor skills, and many experimenters either have tried to control the level of accuracy in their tasks by instructions or have abandoned such tasks in favor of those in which either speed or accuracy is the only criterion of success.

Response Magnitude

The goal for many movements is "as large as possible," such as maximizing height in a high jump or distance in throwing a shot, which has important applications to sport and physical education; surprisingly, they are rarely dealt with in motor skills research. Measurements of such tasks can be in numerous physical units such as amount of force (e.g., strength), distance, or velocity produced.

Secondary Task Methods

Sometimes the above measurements are not particularly revealing, especially when the task is very well learned. For example, measuring driver performance in an automobile in terms of the actual movements the driver makes with the wheel and pedals does not indicate very much about the effects of various independent variables such as the amount of traffic or the level of blood alcohol. Frequently, simultaneous performance on a secondary task, say mental arithmetic, shows changes as a function of independent variables such as traffic load, whereas the actual driving behavior may not. Secondary tasks have been used to study the amount of *attention* required to perform certain acts and are scored in any of the ways described above (e.g., accuracy or speed).

CONSIDERATIONS IN
MEASURING MOTOR LEARNING

Motor learning has been defined in a number of ways by the writers in the field (e.g., Singer, 1968), but to all of them learning is a relatively permanent change in behavior (i.e., motor performance) as a result of experience (i.e., practice) at some activity or task, these changes not representing other processes such as maturation or growth. The idea that the changes are "relatively permanent" rules out the possibility that (1) a performer may improve his score on a particular trial purely by chance and that (2) temporary factors (e.g., drugs) may have improved performance. While this definition is usually accepted without question, there are good reasons why it is inadequate.

Habit Strength

The problem with the definition just stated is that it expresses how learning is *manifested*, but it does not say what learning *is*. Rather, we shall define learning as a relatively permanent change in the internal state of the individual that allows him to perform the motor task in question, and the strength of this internal state is estimated by performance on the motor task. This internal state is a hypothetical construct variously termed *engram*, *associative strength*, *memory trace*, or *habit strength*. Because the term *habit* was the earliest term used in this regard (see James, 1890, chap. 4), it is used here. Therefore, the formal definition to be used in this volume is that *learning is a change, as a result of practice (experience), in a relatively stable internal state termed habit, which is a necessary, but not a sufficient, condition for performance to occur*. The statement that habit is a "necessary" condition for performance means that if habit is not present, the performance cannot occur. That habit is not a "sufficient" condition for performance implies that if habit is present and motivational levels are high and other situational factors are appropriate, performance will occur; otherwise performance might not occur. A good example is fatigue or boredom preventing habit from manifesting itself in performance. Habit, being a hypothetical construct, requires no formal definition in terms of its neurological or biochemical basis. The evidence for habit is that the subject can perform a task after practice that he formerly could not, and this serves as its operational or coordinating definition. Thus, the focus of students of the learning process is on variables that influence the fate of habit.

The increased habit strength (which *is* learning) over practice trials (if we could actually measure it) may not parallel exactly the increased performance (which we *can* measure). For example, the score for the motor task in question may increase rapidly at first, more slowly later, finally approaching an upper limit after many trials. If we could measure directly the habit strength for this task (which we cannot), we *might* find that habit increased linearly with practice trials. (These relationships are plotted in Fig. 3.1.) Actually, we do not have any idea what the form of the gain in habit strength really is, and the guess that it is linear is only one of a great many possibilities. Given these relationships, a number of situations appear to make the original definition of learning unacceptable.

Ceiling and Floor Effects

Ceiling effects are scoring artifacts caused by the fact that the score cannot exceed a certain value. For example, in Fig. 3.1 if the task is scored in percentage correct units, the maximum value of the task, no matter how long the subject practices, is 100 percent. Correspondingly, some tasks have floor effects (e.g., measures of time), with the minimum time being zero

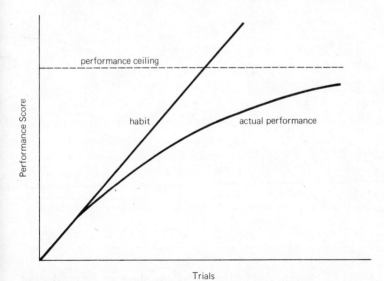

Fig. 3.1 Performance curve of the measured score for the task and the hypothetical function relating the gains in habit strength to practice trials.

seconds or, more realistically, some time below which no
human being could ever perform. If we allow a subject to perform the task beyond the point where he has reached the
ceiling or floor, his scores obviously cannot continue to improve, and we make the conclusion without the notion of
habit that all learning has stopped. But simply because the
score did not change is not evidence that the subject had
stopped learning, since there is evidence that subjects in such
situations continue to improve their speed of responses, do so
with less attention paid to the task, and retain information
better after a period of no practice. Obviously, something was
changing as the subject was practicing at 100 percent correct
and that something is the internal state we term habit.

Temporary Factors

A second problem with the nonhabit definition of learning
concerns a situation in which temporary factors (e.g., fatigue
or boredom) depress performance. Consider Fig. 3.2, in which

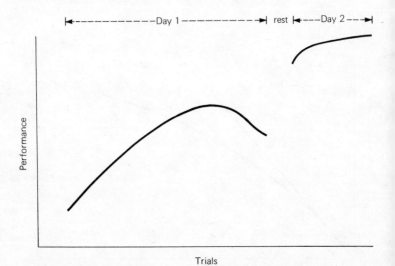

Fig. 3.2 Hypothetical performance curve showing the build-up of
temporary inhibitory factors in original learning. When subjects
are allowed to rest, the inhibitory factors dissipate, and the habit
strength for the task is manifested by improved performance.

subjects are practicing a very boring task for a large number of trials. On the basis of the usual definition of learning, we conclude that subjects learned for awhile, then stopped learning, and then began to forget as practice continued. However, we see that the effect of the boredom was temporary when subjects come back on a second day to perform quite well, as shown by the separate curve on the right. Clearly the subjects, although bored, were learning something during those practice trials, and the learning (i.e., the habit) was not manifested until the boredom was allowed to dissipate through rest.

Methods of Scoring Performance

Many workers have made the statement on the basis of looking at curves such as that in Fig. 3.1 that "learning follows the law of diminishing returns," meaning that the increments in learning are large at first and then become progressively smaller as practice continues or that there is more learning early than late in practice. While it is true that *performance* appears to follow the law of diminishing returns, to say that *learning* does likewise indicates that performance changes are exactly representative of habit strength changes.

This is exemplified by an important methodological paper by Bahrick, Fitts, and Briggs (1957). Their subjects attempted to follow a dot on a screen by moving a hand lever for 9 90-sec trials. After the data had been collected, the experimenters scored the performance in three ways. In one condition, they defined a very narrow area around the correct pathway, and they scored the subject according to how many seconds out of a 90-sec trial that he was in the "correct" area (i.e., "on target"). They did this again for a slightly wider band, and again for a very wide band. When the performances were averaged for all the subjects on each trial separately for each band, and plotted as a function of trials, the curves shown in Fig. 3.3 were produced. The shapes of the performance curves are quite different when the performance is scored in different ways. Using the narrow band (and the inappropriate definition of learning), we conclude that learning is an increasing, *positively* accelerated function of trials; using the medium band, we conclude that the function is linear; and using the wide band, we

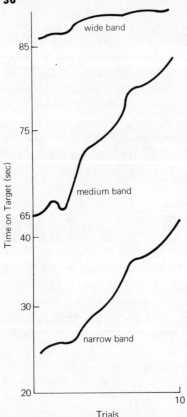

Fig. 3.3 Performance curves for a tracking performance in which the subjects are scored with bands of correctness that are wide, medium, and narrow, producing differently shaped performance curves for the same gains in habit strength. (From Bahrick, Fitts, and Briggs, 1957.)

conclude that the function is *negatively* accelerated. But all of the curves were determined from the *same set of performances*, and therefore the different scoring methods have estimated the same gains in habit strength quite differently. The important point to make here is that if we were not aware that the performance measures were simply *estimates* of habit (learning) *and not in and of themselves learning*, we could have made one conclusion about the form of learning had we used one of the target bands and quite another conclusion had we used another, when in fact there was only *one* pattern of habit strength developed, and the different methods measured it differently. What the actual form of the gain in habit might be is open to question, but looking at one set of curves does not give information about what that form might be.

INDIVIDUAL DIFFERENCES IN LEARNING

The major question concerning individual differences in learning is which of a group of individuals learned the most and which learned the least as a result of practice. "Learning scores" (see Schmidt, 1972a, 1972b) are commonly used, usually the difference in performance between the first few trials and the last few trials; this difference reflects the amount of improvement made in the task as a result of practice. Consider two individuals whose performances are shown in Fig. 3.4. Individual A begins practice with a score of 70 and finishes with a score of 100, giving him a difference score of 30. However, individual B begins with a score of 10 and improves to a score of 80, giving him a difference score of 70. Which person learned more? If learning is simply *changes in performance*, then individual B did. But we argued earlier that learning is a change in *habit strength* estimated by the changes in performance; the question then is which individual gained more habit strength. Since we do not know the relationship between gains in performance and gains in habit, we are not in a position to provide an answer to the question because we are not certain that improving the score from 10 to 80 resulted in more gain in habit strength than did improving the score from 70 to 100. Additionally, ceiling effects could be present in Fig. 3.4, resulting in individual A not being able to "demonstrate" the level of habit strength because of limitation in the scoring system for the task. Therefore, we do not know which of the two individuals learned the most.

However, there are situations in which we *are* able to say which of two individuals learned more: What if individuals A and B started their performance at the same level (say 40) and increased their performance to different levels, to 80 for A and 100 for B. Since the two individuals began with the same

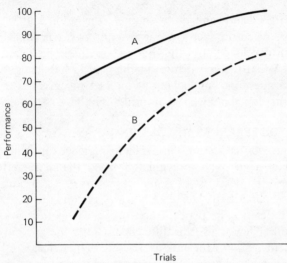

Fig. 3.4 Hypothetical performance curves for two individuals who began practice on the task at different levels and improved to different levels, preventing conclusions about which individual gained the most habit strength.

habit strength and finished with different amounts, the interpretation is that B must have gained more than A and that, therefore, B learned more than A. Thus, statements about the relative amount of gain in habit strength for two individuals can be made meaningfully *only if* their initial performances happen to be equivalent, and this, clearly, will not happen often.

A major problem in classroom grading or evaluation of motor learning bears heavily on the issue of individual differences in learning. It is extremely popular in some circles to "grade on improvement" in motor skills, and the typical method is to give a test at the beginning and at the end of a unit, with the students with the largest *improvement* receiving the highest mark for the unit. This procedure is used because, some feel, final performance is too representative of the amount of "natural ability" possessed by the students; to grade on improvement would allow the person with little ability who improves to receive a high mark without performing as well as a person with high ability. This method of creating learning scores for grading is suspect for many reasons, but the most important reason is that the teacher is attempting to use gains in performance to measure the gains in habit strength. Therefore, while some may prefer "grading on improvement" because of motivation for low-ability students, or for other reasons, the procedure cannot be justified on either methodological or philosophical grounds.

EXPERIMENTS CONCERNING LEARNING

In the "true" experiment (see Chapter 2), the effect of variations in an independent variable on some dependent variable is sought, with the effect of all other variables held constant by appropriate experimental procedures. Frequently in motor skills research an independent variable (e.g., motivating instructions) is varied as subjects are learning a motor task, with performance as the dependent variable (e.g., movement time). Here we might take a group of 100 subjects, randomly divide them into two groups of 50 each, allowing one group (a "control" group, C) to learn under "normal" conditions and the other group (an "experimental" group, E) to learn the task with special motivating instructions. Suppose that we plot

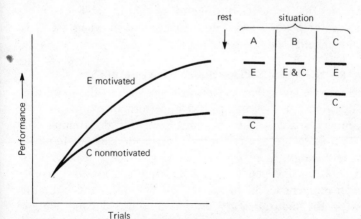

Fig. 3.5 Hypothetical performance curves representing the average performance for two groups practicing under different motivating conditions. Three possible outcomes after the subjects are transferred to nonmotivating conditions are shown in A, B, and C.

the average movement times speed for each of the trials separately for groups C and E, producing the curves in Fig. 3.5. We see that both groups improved somewhat as a result of practice but that the motivated group E improved slightly more. What conclusions should we draw about the effect of the motivating instructions on learning the motor task?

One conclusion that perhaps seems obvious is that subjects in the motivated group *learned more* than the subjects in the nonmotivated group since both groups started at the same performance level (and therefore the same level of habit) and improved to different performance levels. However, in order to be certain that the changes in performance can be attributed to gains in habit strength, we must show that they are "relatively permanent." Therefore, we have two possible explanations for the differences in the left of Fig. 3.5: (1) the motivating instructions created more habit strength, or (2) the motivating instructions exerted a *temporary* (nonhabit) effect on performance (e.g., less boredom). Of course, it is possible that the variable has both effects simultaneously. Independent variables that influence the immediate level of performance but do not affect the gains in habit strength are termed *performance variables. Learning variables* are those independent variables that influence the amount of *gain* in habit strength as a *result* of practice and whose effects remain when the independent variable is removed.

LEARNING VERSUS PERFORMANCE VARIABLES

How do we know that a given variable, such as the motivating instructions in the example, is a performance variable or a learning variable? One convenient way of determining this answer is to use a very simple experimental design termed a *transfer design*. It involves switching the groups to a common level of the independent variable after considerable practice under different levels. In the present example, we could either switch the motivated group to nonmotivated conditions, or switch the nonmotivated group to the motivated condition. If enough time is allowed for the temporary effects (i.e., the motivation, etc.) of the variable to fade away, any differences that remain between the two groups must be due to "relatively permanent" (i.e., habit) effects of the variable, and the variable is a *learning variable*. On the other hand, if all of the difference between the two groups disappears after the switch to common conditions, the differences are due to rather temporary effects, and the variable is a *performance variable*.

The curves to the right of Fig. 3.5 represent the hypothetical performances of the two groups after they had been transferred to common conditions. In situation A, transferring to common conditions produces no effect on the performance, and the variable is a learning variable. In situation B, when the temporary effects of the variable are removed the difference between groups disappears, and the variable is a performance variable. In situation C, the transfer to common conditions results in a partial decrease in the difference between groups, indicating that the variable is both a learning and a performance variable.

As we shall see in Chapter 6, an important task for motor behavior researchers is to classify the various variables that can act during the learning of a motor task into (a) learning variables, (b) performance variables, or (c) both learning and performance variables. This procedure should lead to the more effective structuring of motor learning situations, allowing one to concentrate on variables that are important for learning and to ignore variables that affect performance only temporarily.

CHAPTER 4 WHAT HAPPENS WHEN PEOPLE LEARN?

Since the simple question that serves
as the title of this chapter is really
the central question in motor learning, it is somewhat presumptuous to
devote only one chapter to it. The
question is complex and can be ap-
proached from many points of view.
For example, we might ask how the
individual *performs differently* after
he learns a motor task (as compared
with his performance before). The
answers might be that he performs
more smoothly, with less error, and
so on, which does not describe
a great deal about *how* he has
changed. A more sophisticated approach concerns ways that the subject *organizes himself differently*

after he has learned and usually deals with the way that he uses information he receives from his own body and environment to perform the task more effectively; that is, it concerns the way that responses are chosen, initiated, and controlled. A more complex approach concerns how the *central nervous system* functions and changes in function as a result of learning.

Unfortunately, the large gaps in knowledge between the neurological/biochemical functioning and observable motor behavior do not presently permit an adequate neurological explanation of gross motor learning.[1] As work on this question progresses, however, the two types of analysis will come closer together to aid in the understanding of skill learning. The present chapter describes some of the current thinking in the types of changes that have been referred to earlier as gains in habit.

CHANGES IN OVERALL PERFORMANCE

The most obvious changes that occur as individuals practice is that they generally improve performance on the measures of the task in question. In situations where the performer is provided with information about his performance—either from the experimenter in the form of knowledge of results (KR) or by being able to observe the performance directly—there are generally large improvements in the score that the subject is trying to improve. This, of course, does not *explain* very much about the learning process, but it is the most elementary piece of information that motor behaviorists are attempting to understand. However, what is going on within the individual to produce these changes is a far more interesting and important question.

Occasionally, however, situations will be observed in the laboratory in which subjects do not improve. For example, some very simple reaction-time tasks, in which the performer makes a movement as quickly as he can after a light comes on,

[1] It should not be assumed that an understanding of motor behavior awaits the developments in biochemistry; rather, as Neisser (1967) has said, "Psychology is not just something to do until the biochemist comes. . . ." A behavioral understanding is necessary to the development of neurological principles, and vice versa.

and simple limb-speed tasks show improvements only for a trial or two, and then performance tends to level off. Generally, as the task becomes more and more complicated (in that more strange or awkward movements are required) the period over which improvement occurs lengthens. Additionally, tasks whose scoring system is insensitive to gains in habit strength because of, for example, ceiling effects cannot show improved performance with practice.

THE LIMITS OF PERFORMANCE

One often hears such statements as "It took me 20 minutes to learn to ride my bicycle," implying that learning was finished after 20 minutes, with no further improvements in performance taking place after this time. Actually, there is a great deal of evidence to suggest that learning is never finished. For example, Snoddy (1926) has shown that subjects who practiced a task in which they drew figures while seeing only the mirror image of their hand continued to improve over 100 days of practice. Also, Crossman (1959) has provided data from factory workers who used a small jig to make cigars indicating that time required per cigar continued to decrease over 7 years of practice, representing some 10 million cigars! To be sure, the improvements were not large after the first large gains, but they were present nevertheless and indicated that the learning may *never* be completed. Subjective observations from champion athletes also seem to suggest that learning may continue for many years.

In other situations there are, beyond initial improvements, no obvious changes in the main performance score for a task; a good example is driving performance. However, if the level of learning is measured by alternative measures such as the amount of attention required for the task (skill in performing a secondary task at the same time), it can usually be shown that individuals do, in fact, continue to perform better in terms of the amount of effort and muscular tension needed to perform the tasks. Therefore, there is really no evidence to suggest that learning stops after a certain number of trials and considerable evidence to suggest that learning is a never-ending, continuous process.

THE STAGES OF LEARNING

There is some evidence to suggest that as the performer practices he passes through a number of stages in the way he performs. One way to envision these different stages was proposed
by Fitts and Posner (1967), and it is presented here in brief
version. Of course, such phases of performance are not marked
by clear boundaries, but are rather gradual changes that seem
to differentiate one level of performance from another.

Cognitive Phase

In the early part of learning any new motor skill, the primary
problem to the performer seems to be to understand the motor
problem and what is to be done. He needs to know in general
terms how the apparatus operates, how the task is scored, and
what he is to accomplish. The performer then engages in considerable cognitive activity, including making strategies about
what he will try to do to maximize his score, trying to remember how he attacked similar problems in the past, and so on.
Usually the first attempt will not be particularly successful,
and he will engage in additional cognitive activity to ready
himself for the next attempt. In the cognitive phase the performer makes use of his immense verbal, or reasoning, capacity
to attempt to solve the motor problem. Inappropriate strategies
are discarded in a few trials, and more appropriate ones are
retained; he learns what he can do with the apparatus and
what he cannot, and he does not attempt to manipulate the
apparatus in inappropriate ways after the first few attempts at
it. At the same time, there is large improvement in the performance scores, the major changes being in deciding which movements to make rather than how to make a given movement
more efficiently or effectively. Because of the great use of the
intellectual capacities in this stage, Adams (1971) has termed
this stage the *verbal-motor stage*.

Associative Phase

This phase has been termed the *motor stage* by Adams to describe the dropping out of initial cognitive activities and refin-
ing the necessary motor movements. The performer does not
make large errors in his responses during this stage, and he

gradually attempts to improve his responses without actually changing them a great deal, as he would in the cognitive stage. Also, during this stage the performer begins to be able to recognize when he has made an error in his response without having to be told about the error from the experimenter or teacher; he can correct those errors very quickly and efficiently via an *error detection mechanism*. In the associative stage, the problem for the individual shifts from the "what to do" of the previous phase to "how to do it."

Autonomous Phase

This third phase describes extremely advanced levels of performance after a great deal of practice. In addition to the efficient responding, greatly reduced errors, and high rates of working, performers seem to become more "automatic" in making their responses. In one sense, the responses require less *attention*, and "spare attention" can be devoted to other tasks that can be performed simultaneously. A good example is driving a car, a task in which nearly full attention is required in early practice and greatly reduced attention when the individual has been driving for a number of years; he is free to think of the events of the day, to carry on conversations, and so on, while driving, and with minimal impairment in the responses involved in controlling the vehicle. In another sense the performer becomes able to carry out longer and longer segments of behavior when previously each of the elements had to be performed separately. For example, the skilled typist can type whole words or even groups of words in one "act" while the novice types one letter at a time. As important as the autonomous phase seems for the understanding of human motor skills and their learning, researchers seldom deal with skills that are learned to such advanced levels; limitations in time, subject availability, and funds for research have legislated in favor of performances falling in the associative stage.

OLD HABITS BECOME NEW SKILLS

One interesting hypothesis about motor skills learning is that all motor learning is really over by a very early age (about 4 years). It is assumed that during these early years the performer acquires a repertoire of basic movements. Some researchers see these movements as jumping, hopping, skipping, balancing, throwing, and so on, while others see them as being even smaller, such as moving the arm in a number of ways, grasping, and following objects with the head and eyes. In either case, the idea is that these basic movements form "building blocks" for the more complex movements that are learned by children and young adults. Thus "new" movements (e.g., pole vaulting) are not seen as new but as a combination of "old" movements in some new way. It should be recognized that although there is considerable popular support for this hypothesis, there is very little research evidence to support it, and it would be very difficult to determine if this idea is really correct. The basic movement concept is important to physical education, as many curricula for elementary physical education are based on the assumption that old movements recombine into new movements. An opposing view, the "specificity of learning" idea presented by Henry (1968) and his students, says that all learning, even at older ages, consists of learning *new* motor patterns that are not dependent on the so-called basic movements.

HIERARCHICAL CONTROL THEORY

The hierarchical control theory is based on the idea that the motor system is structured *hierarchically*, with certain structures having rather broad responsibilities for the operation of the entire system, having control over "lower" subsystems that carry out specific functions. One such model of human performance, proposed by Fitts (1964), uses the idea that there is an *executive* responsible for seeing to it that certain motor responses are carried out. The executive "surveys" the motor problem to be solved, selects the appropriate motor movements to be produced, and sends "instructions" to have them executed. At this point, control is shifted to a lower system, usually termed the *effector*, which actually carries out these instructions. The effector is usually seen as a set of *motor programs*, which when activated produces commands to the muscles that produce the movement. The analogy to the electronic computer is clear. The executive is the computer programmer who senses the need to accomplish a task and then writes a program to instruct the machine as to the actions to take to solve the problem. Once the program is written, the executive transfers his control to the program and the instructions written therein are carried out faithfully, even if the instructions may have been inappropriate. After the program has finished its operation, the results of the activities are fed back to the executive for checking, and the control now resides with the executive again. He can decide to use the existing program and results, or, if an error has been made, he can rewrite the program, shifting control once again to the effector for action. The information about the correctness of the outcome of the effector's actions is termed *feedback*, and it serves as the basis for future actions by the executive.

Fitts saw the roles of the effector and executive changing somewhat as the performer learns the motor task. At first, the motor programs for action are not well developed, and the executive does not rely on them heavily. Rather, the executive "orders" single movements and checks the outcome of each action as frequently as it can. Such procedures are relatively inefficient and result in responding that is characteristic of the "jerky" performances of novices. After a great deal of practice, however, the learner refines and extends the motor programs, and the executive relies more and more heavily on them to produce the movements. Thus, the executive transfers more of the control to the effector, which carries out longer and longer strings of actions. The executive begins to monitor the outcome of these strings of actions rather than each of the actions making up the string, with the result that attention of the executive is freed to perform other tasks. When the individual is performing in the autonomous phase of learning, nearly all of the control lies with the effector, and the executive needs to pay very little attention to the feedback from the task.

Pew (1966) has provided some support for this theory in an experiment in which subjects pressed two buttons, one with each hand, to control movements of a dot on a screen. When the right-hand button was pressed, the dot accelerated to the right, and when the left-hand button was pressed the dot accelerated to the left, and the subjects' job was to press the buttons in such a way that the dot remained centered in the screen. In the early stages of practice, subjects adopted a strategy in which they pressed one button and waited for the dot to react so that they could see the error developing directly; then they made another button press depending on where the dot was at that later time. Because subjects made from two to three presses per second, the performances were quite jerky and subjects were largely unsuccessful in keeping the dot centered on the screen. However, after a great deal of practice, the subjects adopted a different strategy wherein they pressed the buttons very rapidly in alternation with a rate of about eight per second. It appeared as though the subjects were programming about five button presses at once, observing the error and correcting it every second or so by modifying the pattern of finger movements (i.e., by holding one button down slightly longer than the other). In terms of the theory, in early practice the executive was in control of every response, and error from each response had to be fed back before the next response could be made, leading to very jerky performances. However, in later practice, the executive shifted the control to the effector mechanism and allowed the movements to be carried out for a greater period of time before the executive had to exert control to change the pattern of movements.

A word of caution is in order. Fitts did not really say that there are such things in the body as executives and effectors, and that they work in the way specified above; rather, he made an *analogy*, or model (see Chapter 2), stating that the individual seems to perform *as if* there were such structures present. Seen in this light, the model really does not explain how individuals learn, but it is useful for providing a way of thinking about the process by showing how it is similar to other processes with which we are familiar, such as the operation of a computer.

CHANGING COMPONENT ABILITIES

Another way that the learning process can be viewed uses the concept of the *ability*, a term that most of us have heard but that is rarely used properly. An ability is a hypothetical construct (see Chapter 2) that refers to a general trait of the individual, inferred from performances on certain kinds of tasks. If an individual can perform a number of tasks very well, all of which require him to react quickly when a light comes on (e.g., with the finger, the leg), we say that the individual has a good *ability* to react. Abilities are thought to be rather constant over time, some being present at birth (e.g., color vision) and others being developed somewhat during childhood. The term *ability* should be differentiated from the term *skill*, which refers to the level of performance in a single task only. More will be said about skill and ability in Chapter 9.

The most important idea about the relationship between abilities and practice comes from Fleishman (1965), who believes that a given motor task has underlying it a number of motor and cognitive abilities. For example, hitting a baseball successfully seems to require the ability to anticipate upcoming events, to move rapidly, to react quickly to changes in the environment, and so on. Further, Fleishman believes that the pattern of abilities important for a given task in very early practice is different from the pattern in later practice; that is, the pattern of abilities changes as practice continues. For example, performance in the first few practice trials might be heavily dependent on "cognitive" abilities, whereas in later practice the performance might be dependent on more "motor" abilities.

Another way to think of this process is in terms of the *changes in the task* as the individual practices it. It is possible to describe a task in terms of the abilities required and the relative importance of each. If the pattern of abilities changes with practice, we can say that the *task* is not the same task early in practice as it is later in practice. Of course, the apparatus and scoring procedures are identical, but the make-up of the abilities that underlie it is different, so that the task might be considered a different task between early and late practice.

Fleishman and Rich (1963) allowed subjects to practice 10 trials on a task called the two-hand coordination test, in which subjects had to move two crank handles (one with each hand) to control the movement of a pointer to follow a moving target. Subjects performed two additional tests. One of these was termed *kinesthetic sensitivity* and involved the ability to judge small weights lifted with the hand. The second measure was a paper-and-pencil test to determine the ability to orient oneself in space. Fleishman and Rich then plotted performance on the motor task separately for subjects who were classified "high" or "low" on the kinesthetic sensitivity measure, and the curves are shown in Fig. 4.1 (top). The ability to judge weights was not important early in practice on the task, as shown by the fact that subjects with low and high kinesthetic sensitivity were about the same in motor task performance on the first trial; but in later practice, subjects high in kinesthetic sensitivity were superior to the subjects low in that measure, indicating that some ability related to the weight judgments was also important to performance of the motor task in later practice.

The same analysis was completed with the spatial measure. Subjects who were high on the spatial measure performed trial 1 of the task more proficiently than subjects low on that measure, but these differences were not present in later practice (Fig. 4.1, bottom). These data indicate that abilities underlying the task in early practice were not present in later practice, and vice versa, supporting the idea that the pattern of abilities for the task had changed with practice. A similar study with essentially the same conclusions was conducted earlier by Fleishman and Hempel (1954).

Knowing that abilities underlying the task change with practice is very important from practical points of view. For example, assume that I choose my starting team on the basis of performance on the first practice session before much learning had taken place. In this case I might be measuring abilities present in early practice that are not representative of abilities required for later in the season. Thus, a student who is quite poor on the first trial might lack the abilities necessary to perform at this level of practice but might be the best performer after extensive practice because the task might then depend on abilities that the individual did have. Selecting on the basis of early performance could result in inefficient selection of the starting team.

INCREASED AUTOMATIZATION WITH PRACTICE

Automaticity has two rather different meanings for motor skills. One meaning is that the accomplished subject is able to pay less *attention* to his performance as it is going on than is

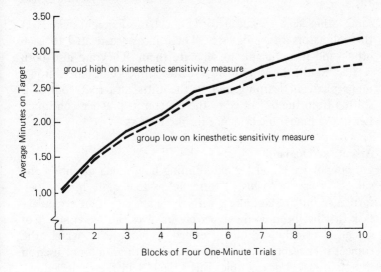

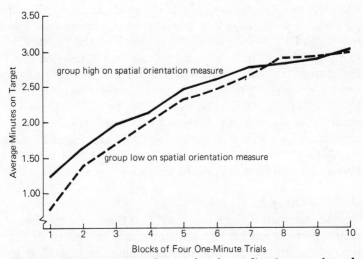

Fig. 4.1 Performance on the two-hand coordination test for subjects classified high versus low on kinesthetic sensitivity and high versus low on spatial orientation. (From Fleishman and Rich, 1963.)

the novice, thus freeing the former either to perform other tasks or to concentrate on different aspects of the main task. A second meaning is that one set of mechanisms might be involved in the movement control in early practice, but that some other (more "automatic") mechanism might take over this job as practice progresses. These ideas are related to each other, and it is difficult to separate them. They are also both related to the ideas presented earlier concerning the autonomous phase of learning and to the Fitts idea that control is shifted from the executive to the effector as practice continues. Let us examine some evidence for these views.

Attention Demand

One popular method for determining how much attention the subject is paying to his performance is to require him to perform a secondary task along with the main task. One secondary task that has been used extensively involves the presentation of a signal, usually auditory (termed a *probe*), to which the subject is to react as quickly as possible with a limb not used in the main task. For example, Ells (1969) had the subject move a pointer to a target as quickly as he could after a signal and presented a probe at various locations in the movement. The subject had to make a left-finger response to the probe. Ells found that as practice continued in this simple task the reaction time to the probe decreased, implying that the main movement was becoming more automatic and freeing the attention capacities of the subject to react to the probe. Very similar results have been found recently by Salmoni (1973). Thus, there is evidence that the attention required of subjects as they perform a motor task decreases with practice, at least as attention is measured by such probe techniques.

Shifts to Other Mechanisms

Another automaticity hypothesis says that the responses become more automatic not because less attention is demanded during the movements, but because the controlling functions shift to other mechanisms. This is what is implied in the Fitts hierarchical control theory, where the shift is from executive (decision-making) processes to effector (motor) processes. Bahrick and Shelley (1954) showed this effect quite well. Their subjects watched a screen with a horizontal slit, behind which came dots in 10 columns. In one condition the dots appeared in a very regular pattern so that after some practice the subjects could predict which dot would appear next; in the other condition the subjects could not make this prediction. Each subject's job was to press one of 10 keys, pairing his fingers and thumbs to each column of dots, at the moment each dot appeared; the subject also had to perform mental arithmetic. Bahrick and Shelley argued that increased automatization of the button-pressing task would allow superior performance in mental arithmetic. When the task was regular and predictable, practice greatly increased the subjects' skill in mental arithmetic, implying that the main task control had been shifted to the timing or prediction mechanisms, but the irregular task showed no such improvements in mental arithmetic. The interpretation is that other mechanisms developed as a result of practice are able to perform activities that the decision-making process must assume in early practice and that this frees the decision-making mechanisms to perform other tasks.

ERROR DETECTION MECHANISMS

Another way that the individual changes with practice is in his increasing capability for detecting errors in his responses and ability to correct them more quickly as well. A number of theoretical statements have been made about how such error detection mechanisms might operate and how they develop over the course of practice. (See Adams, 1971.) There is considerable evidence that subjects do develop such mechanisms, and one of these investigations is presented below.

Schmidt and White (1972) had subjects learn a very simple task in which they tried to move a slide a distance of 9 inches in exactly 150 msec (0.15 sec). Immediately following each attempt, subjects reported what they thought their score was on the just-completed trial, and then the experimenter gave them their actual score for that trial. Schmidt and White examined the correlation (within subjects) between what a subject said he did (subjective score) and what he actually did (objective score) as a measure of the strength of the error detection mechanism; a plot of this score is shown in Fig. 4.2. The subjects became increasingly sensitive to the direction and magnitude of their errors over the course of two days' practice, as indicated by the progressively increasing correlations shown in Fig. 4.2. In addition, at the end of practice the mean difference between objective and subjective scores was only 7 msec, showing the subjects' remarkable accuracy in being able to guess their own scores.

This evidence supports the notion that the subjects developed a capacity to determine their own errors on the basis of a learned internal error detection mechanism and that these mechanisms were remarkably accurate. The fact that they are developed with practice supports the notion that the individual could use his own error information (from his error detection mechanism) as a substitute for knowledge of results (KR); this effect has been termed *subjective reinforcement*. The obvious advantage of subjective reinforcement is that learners are capable of providing their *own* KR so that learning can continue even when the experimenter (or teacher) is not present.

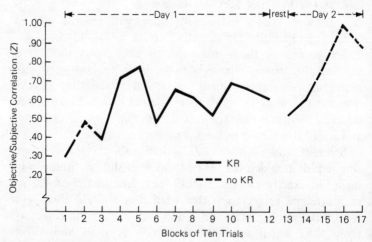

Fig. 4.2 Mean correlation (Z) between objective (actual) and subjective (estimated) error as a function of practice. (From Schmidt and White, 1972.)

CHAPTER 5 | THE TRANSFER OF LEARNING

Traditionally, transfer of learning has been defined as a gain (or loss) in performance on one task as a result of practice on some other task. However, for the same reasons cited in Chapter 3 concerning the concept of learning, it will be preferable to define transfer as the gain (or loss) in *habit strength* for one task as a result of practicing another task, with those habit gains being estimated by the gains or losses in *performance* for the task. Practice on one task may result in *gains* in habit strength for another task (positive transfer) or *losses* in habit strength (negative transfer). The transfer of learning is usually an unseen factor in learning motor skills. It was mentioned in Chapter 4 that motor learning after a very young age might not involve learning new skills, but rather consist of a recombination of old skills into "new" motor patterns. Thus the adult's job in learning a new motor skill might consist of *transferring* those old skills to the new situation.

THE MEASUREMENT OF TRANSFER

The measurement of transfer presents many of the same problems found in the measurement of habit strength, discussed in Chapter 3. There are a number of experimental designs to evaluate transfer effects, but the most simple concerns the use of two experimental groups:

	Transfer Task	*Criterion Task*
Group I	left-hand task	right-hand task
Group II	nothing	right-hand task

For example, assume that group I has 50 trials of practice on a left-hand movement-time task (transfer task) and then has 50 trials on a different right-hand movement-time task (criterion task). How much did the left-hand task transfer to the right-hand task? We can answer this question by using a control group, group II, which has practice only on the right-hand task, so that the only way in which the groups differ is whether or not they have had experience with the left-hand task. Therefore the difference between the groups in the right-hand performance for the first few trials will represent the degree of transfer from left to right. This is illustrated in Fig. 5.1 (left side), in which the performances of the two groups *on the right-hand task* are plotted. Notice that group I, which has had the experience with the left-hand task before attempting the right-hand task, performs better initially than does group II, which did not have the left-hand practice; this difference in performance is taken as evidence that the left-hand task transferred to the right-hand task. The transfer is positive since the left-hand task improved the right. Contrast this with the right

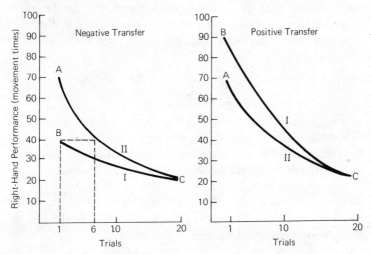

Fig. 5.1 Hypothetical performance curves showing positive transfer and negative transfer.

side of Fig. 5.1, showing that the left-hand task *interfered* with the right-hand task. Here the initial performance of group I is worse than that of group II, indicating that the experience on the left-hand task was detrimental to performance on the left-hand task, an example of *negative* transfer.

The amount of transfer in experiments with the above paradigm is usually estimated on the first few trials of the task. The performance on trial 1 is a good measure of the amount of transfer from some other task. This is preferred to using a number of trials because including later trails brings in the amount of transfer from the other task as well as the learning of the task that occurred on trial 1. Therefore, using as few trials as possible at the beginning of the task will provide the most sensitive measure of the amount of transfer. There are many ways to quantify transfer in experiments such as those reported above; two of the most important are presented below.

Percentage Transfer
The percentage transfer is estimated by the gain in performance of the transferred group (I) over its control group (II) on the first criterion task trial, divided by the total amount of

improvement that the control group experiences in the criterion task. For example, using the curves presented in Fig. 5.2, we can measure the percentage transfer by this formula:

$$\text{Percentage Transfer} = \frac{A - B}{A - C} \times 100$$

We see that the percentage transfer in the present example is $(70 - 40)/(70 - 20) \times 100 = 60$ percent. This means that 60 percent of the improvement in the right-hand task was gained by practicing the left-hand task. In the case of negative transfer we see that the formula is $(70 - 90)/(70 - 20) \times 100 = -20/50 = 40$ percent *negative* transfer, meaning that the right-hand task caused ⅔ as much decrement in the task as there was improvement by the control group.

Savings Score
A second, less popular method for measuring transfer is the savings score. We notice from Fig. 5.1 (left) that group I began practicing the task at a point equivalent to the level of group II on the sixth trial, and we say that there was a savings score of six trials. This means that six trials of right-hand practice were "saved" by practicing the left-hand task first.

Problems in Measuring Transfer
Both of these methods for measuring transfer have a number of methodological problems related to the fact that when inferences about internal processes (such as gains in habit) are made from measures of performance, we are confronted with all of the problems inherent in measuring habit discussed in Chapter 3. Performance curves are sensitive not only to gains in habit strength, but also to temporary factors such as fatigue or boredom, and the measured amount of transfer can be altered considerably by changing the conditions of practice. Transfer is also sensitive to the amount of practice given to the control group, since increasing the amount of learning increases the denominator of the ratio and would decrease the measured

percentage transfer. Thus the measurement of transfer is quite arbitrary, and great care must be taken in interpreting the results of transfer experiments.

THE TYPES OF TRANSFER

Transfer can occur in a number of different situations, and for convenience they are subdivided into a number of categories. *Intertask transfer* is concerned with transfer from one task to another, such as from tennis to swimming, while *intratask transfer* is concerned with transfer from one variation of a task to another, such as from driving one car to driving another. *Part-whole transfer* is concerned with transfer from a part of a task to the whole task, such as from learning to toss the tennis ball (only) on a serve to the total serve including the toss.

Intertask Transfer

There is not a great deal of evidence on intertask transfer. However, a few studies have been conducted to determine to what extent practicing activities designed to develop "quickness" might transfer to other tasks in which "quickness" was important. Blankenship (1952) and Lindeburg (1949) had subjects perform special "quickening exercises" in class situations, and the possible transfer to a task that required them to react and move quickly was measured. In neither study was there a transfer effect, either positive or negative, from the exercises to the motor task requiring quickness.

More generally, it is believed that if task A requires some ability (like quickness or steadiness), practicing another task B that also uses this ability will improve task A because task B "developed" the ability. The evidence from Blankenship and Lindeburg does not support this notion, and there is little evidence that such general intertask transfer effects are possible. Also, abilities (see Chapters 4 and 9) are thought to be innate and not modifiable by practice; thus no changes in such abilities should be expected from this practice, leaving no learning to transfer to the first task.

Intertask transfer is present in other situations, however,

as Woodward (1943) has found; assembly-line workers had to assemble two objects with similar operations and numbers of parts, but with parts of different shapes. There was small positive transfer (about 5 percent) between the two tasks. This transfer could have been the result of the similar *order* of operations between the two tasks, however, and might not have been the result of transfer of "motor" skill.

Another question that students frequently ask about transfer concerns the extent to which practice on a game of one type might transfer (either positively or negatively) to another game of the same type (e.g., tennis and badminton). There is very little good evidence on this question, but from what we know about intratask transfer (see next section), it would appear that such transfer is negligible. Of course, as the elements of the game become more similar (e.g., handball and paddleball), because of the type of court or implement used, there might be more positive transfer. Also, there is *no* evidence that practicing one skill transfers *negatively* to (i.e., interferes with) the learning of some other task of the same type.

Many individuals feel that certain *patterns* of movement —a good example is the so-called overarm pattern used in throwing—are learned in one task and are transferable to other tasks that presumably use the "same" pattern, but there is little evidence for this view. It appears that the patterns, although they outwardly appear to use the same muscular actions for various tasks (e.g., throwing versus hitting a handball), are actually quite different and require learning and practice on each task separately. This is in keeping with the ideas of Henry (1968), who believes that even very similar-appearing motor skills are probably based on very different patterns of muscular activity. It is hardly strange, therefore, that two tasks such as tennis and badminton may not transfer to one another.

In summary, intertask motor transfer is *never* negative and is usually quite low-positive unless the tasks have obvious "cognitive" elements in common with one another. There is no research evidence that abilities may be developed on one task to be transferred to another using that ability, nor is there research evidence of the transfer of "basic movement patterns" from task to task.

Intratask Transfer

There has been a great deal of research conducted concerning transfer from one variation of a task to another variation of the same task, here termed *intratask transfer*. Since the results seem to depend on the type of task studied, the basic classifications of tasks are treated in turn.

Continuous tasks. Lordahl and Archer (1958) used the pursuit rotor task, in which the subject attempted to follow with a hand-held stylus a target that moved in a circular path, and studied the transfer among various speeds of rotation. Three groups practiced at either 40, 60, or 80 rpm for 30 trials and then transferred to the 60-rpm task for additional trials. They found that transfer was positive in all cases, ranging from 12 percent to 31 percent. Namikas and Archer (1960) used the same procedures and found that transfer ranged from 42 percent to 64 percent. Other studies using tracking tasks have found that transfer from one version of the task to another was in the same general range, from 22 percent to 58 percent. The extent of transfer found in these studies might at first seem large, but it should be remembered that all of these studies have investigated transfer among tasks that were very similar; in fact, the only difference between the transfer and criterion tasks were simple changes in speed of target movement or of the sensitivity of the controls, using the same apparatus. In view of the fact that the transfer was usually less than 50 percent, one is forced to the conclusion that the amount of motor transfer is generally quite small.

Lordahl and Archer also studied the transfer among various target sizes and among various target speeds, showing that the transfer among sizes was somewhat larger (54 percent) than the transfer among speeds (12 percent and 31 percent). These data might imply that transfer is greater if the spatial (e.g., target size) components of the task are varied, leaving the timing (or rhythm) components of the task intact, than if the rhythm or speed of the task is varied, holding the spatial aspects constant. Taken cautiously, these data would suggest that the rhythmic (or timing) components of the tasks should be as similar as possible if transfer among the tasks is to be maximized and might suggest that "slow-motion" practice of sports skills is not as effective as practice at full speed.

Discrete tasks. There is not very much evidence concerning transfer among discrete tasks; thus the conclusions about this area of transfer are not very clear. Szafran and Welford (1950) used two methods of tossing small loops of chain at a target, either tossing them directly or "lobbing" them over a bar. They found only 14 percent transfer between the two methods of tossing, indicating that quite different patterns of movement were developed in the two tasks. In contrast, Schmidt (1968) studied a task in which the subject had to release his hand from a key, move to knock over three barriers in a right-center-left order, and return his hand to the key as quickly as possible. Schmidt varied the task to produce four slightly different tasks by changing the locations (but not the order) of the barriers. The experimental group (group E) practiced tasks 1, 2, 3, and 4 (40 trials of each), while the control group (group C) practiced only task 4. The performances of the groups on task 4 are shown in Fig. 5.2. The transfer from tasks 1–3 to task 4 was nearly complete, with group E beginning practice at almost the same level of performance as group C reached after 40 trials; transfer was computed to be 93 percent. Here is a clear case of the large positive transfer that can occur between similar skills, and the transfer effect remains after a 24-hr lay-off on day 2. Thus, it must be concluded that transfer among discrete skills may be extremely large if the tasks are sufficiently similar, but need not be, as seen in Szafran and Welford's experiment above. In addition, there was no evidence of negative transfer among discrete skills.

Relative task difficulty. One of the most-asked questions about transfer is whether it is more beneficial for transfer to learn a difficult task first followed by an easy task, or vice versa. This question has received a great deal of research attention. Typically, experimenters have made one version of the motor task more "difficult" by changing the speed of a target, decreasing the size of targets to be followed or struck, increasing the distance over which subjects propel objects to strike a

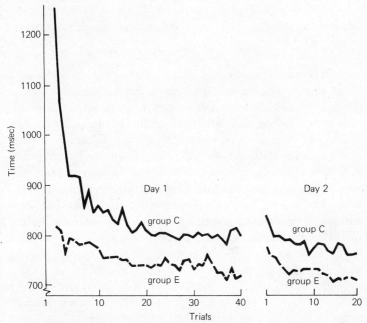

Fig. 5.2 Evidence for transfer in a discrete motor task. Mean movement time on task 4 for group C with no prior practice and group E with prior practice on tasks 1, 2, and 3. (From Schmidt, 1968.)

target (e.g., in archery), and so on. In an unpublished review of the literature on transfer of learning by Schmidt (1966), nearly the same number of studies supported the easy-to-difficult order as superior as supported the difficult-to-easy order, and many studies reported no differences in the amount of transfer for the two methods. The entire area of research is quite confused, and it seems safe to say that the answer to the question is not known. A major problem has been that there is no adequate definition of *difficulty* that can be applied to all motor tasks. Traditionally, if some variable decreases performance on a motor task, it is said that the task under these conditions is "more difficult." Since a great number of experimental variables can influence motor performance, and hence by definition affect difficulty, there is little wonder that difficulty, as defined in the literature, bears no systematic relationship to transfer. The entire concept of difficulty needs to be rethought.

Part-to-Whole Transfer

Tasks can be divided into parts in a number of ways so that the individuals can learn the parts separately, with the intent of later integrating the parts to form the whole task again. In serial tasks (e.g., learning to start a car) the division into parts may be quite "natural," with the parts being easily recognized as separate. In other tasks, however, the division is often not natural, such as practicing the leg and arm movements separately in learning to swim or practicing the backswing separately from the downswing in a golf shot. The research dealing with the effectiveness of such part-whole transfer has provided mixed findings, probably because of the wide variety of tasks used. The various types of task are discussed below.

Serial tasks. Using a serial industrial task with a number of separate operations on a lathe, Seymour (1954) found that part practice was superior to whole practice, probably because the "easy" operations were learned quickly and had to be repeated each time in whole practice, while the "difficult" operations could be practiced in isolation in the part practice. Also, Adams and Hufford (1962) found that learning a series of discrete acts that were part of the total task of flying an airplane transferred greatly to those operations in the whole task. Therefore, when the total task involves a set of rather separate and independent actions, which are not to be performed at the same time (i.e., they are not "time shared"), it seems profitable to divide the task into its components for isolated part practice.

Continuous tasks. In tracking tasks and other continuous performances, investigators have divided multicomponent tasks into parts by providing practice on one of the components separately. Briggs and Brogden (1954) and Briggs and Waters (1958) used a lever-positioning task that required positioning in two dimensions (forward/backward and right/left) and found that practice on the dimensions separately transferred to the whole task. However, some tasks have components that *interact*—that is, manipulating one of the components requires an adjustment of another component. In swimming the crawl stroke, a less forceful stroke requires a greater head turn in order to breathe. In such situations, attempting to transfer the parts to the whole does not appear to be very successful, probably because the learner needs to have the parts presented together so that he can learn how they interact and how to deal with them. Speaking practically, if there is a great deal of interaction among components, the task will probably be learned more efficiently if the task is not split into components for learning.

Discrete tasks. There is little evidence on part practice for discrete tasks, but a study by Lersten (1968) provides a great deal of insight into the problem. Lersten's subjects had to make a circular movement of a hand-operated handle followed by a linear movement to knock over a small barrier; the total movement resembled a rho (ρ). Lersten provided practice on either the circular component or the linear component in isolation and studied the transfer of these parts to the whole task. He found that practice on the isolated components was nearly ineffective in producing transfer to the whole task, with some part practice even producing *negative* transfer to the whole! It was clear that the part-to-whole practice procedures neither developed additional skill for the total task nor saved practice time.

It is sometimes dangerous to conclude too much from only one investigation, but Lersten's findings suggest that discrete skills do not lend themselves to part practice. It may be that the division of the usually short (in time) discrete skills is too arbitrary and "unnatural," so that the subject is practicing a part that is not the same as that part in the context of the total skill. It also may be that simultaneously performed parts of a discrete skill interact considerably, so that practice on one part in isolation does not provide learning about the interaction of that part and the other parts in the skill. It would seem, then, that dividing discrete skills into parts, a practice that we see frequently in physical education classes, may be ineffective when the division is unnatural or when the parts have a high degree of interdependence.

Negative Transfer

The question of possible negative transfer in motor learning situations is important from theoretical points of view, but it is especially important from practical points of view. If we are producing decrements in performance on some tasks at the same time that we are providing learning on others, the net effect at the end of a semester of practice could be quite small in terms of the total amount of habit gained.

Very few investigations concerning negative transfer in motor learning have been made, but a landmark study was conducted some time ago by Lewis, McAllister, and Adams (1951). They used the Mashburn task, a three-dimensional, continuous tracking task, with independent dimensions being the right-left position of foot pedals and the forward-backward and right-left position of an aircraft-type control stick. A display provided information about the locations of each of the three control dimensions. "Target" locations of the controls could also be presented on the display, and the subject's job was to position the controls so that each control position matched the corresponding target location. When all three dimensions were aligned, the subject was said to have made a "match," and then a new set of targets would appear and the subject would attempt another "match," and so on, the score being the number of matches in a 2-min trial. A "standard" task involved movements of the display indicator in the same direction as the movements of the controls (e.g., pressing the right foot pedal moved the display indicator to the right), and a "reversed" task involved opposite movements (e.g., pushing the right pedal moved the indicator to the *left*).

Lewis et al. provided practice on either 10, 30, or 50 original learning (OL) trials of the standard task, shifted to the reversed task for either 10, 20, 30, or 50 interpolated learning (IL) trials, and then resumed practice on the standard task. The amount of negative transfer (or interference) was measured by the decrease in performance from the end of the first standard task performance to the beginning of the standard task after the reversed task practice and thus indicated the amount of negative transfer that was caused by practice on the reversed task. The results of the experiment are shown in Fig. 5.3. As can be seen, there was considerable negative transfer, and the negative transfer increased as the amount of IL (reversed task practice) increased. Also, as the number of OL trials increased, there was an increased amount of negative transfer, as seen by the upward slope of all the curves in Fig. 5.3. The Lewis et al. study and an additional one by McAllister (1952) are the only studies that show clear evidence of negative transfer in motor learning.

As we have seen before, transfer from task to task is nearly always positive but low in value, and the interpretation was that there were some similarities between the tasks that allowed

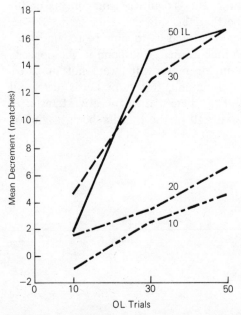

Fig. 5.3 Relationship between amount of original learning (OL) on the standard task and amount of interpolated learning (IL) on the reversed task on the Mashburn apparatus. (From Lewis, McAllister, and Adams, 1951.)

them to transfer positively. However, Lewis et al. went to great lengths to make the tasks *opposite* from one another; that is, the response that was learned to one stimulus situation in the standard task was exactly opposite to that required in the reversed task. Apparently, tasks have to be this different— different to the point of being opposite or contradictory— before negative transfer can occur. Unless there are clearly opposite (not simply different) responses required for a given stimulus situation, the transfer among tasks will be small but positive. This might imply that the transfer among various sports should be positive and that teachers needn't worry about producing negative transfer among sport skills so long as they do not have their students learning clearly contradictory responses.

The Lewis et al. study is not a clear-cut demonstration of negative transfer in *motor learning* since it can be argued that what was transferred were the "cognitive" components of the task. Thus, it could be that the subjects, after facing the reversed task, simply were confused as to how to respond (i.e., what to do), and once they learned to respond in the opposite direction their actual motor movements were not impaired. We have no way of determining this from Lewis' data, but there is the possibility that there was no negative transfer of *motor learning* at all, with all of the transfer being cognitive.

CHAPTER 6

THE CONDITIONS OF PRACTICE

This chapter deals with topics that were the primary concern of the field of motor skills during the period from 1930 to 1955 or so and treats the factors and variables that operate within a practice session to influence the performance and/or learning of motor skills. Most of this work was done with practical application in mind, as the concern for how to best structure learning settings for physical education classes, pilot training, and industrial training was an important consideration. As mentioned in Chapter 1, this emphasis has shifted somewhat toward research leading to a basic understanding of motor performance and learning, with a strong emphasis on theories of motor learning and human performance. However, because the variables influencing practice and learning are still important, some of them are treated in this chapter.

VARIABLES ACTING BEFORE ACTUAL PRACTICE
Instructions
The instructions given to the learners of motor tasks are usually considered to be a very important determiner of the outcome of the learning experience. It is generally believed (e.g., Singer, 1972, p. 273) that instructions should be rather simple at first, become more complex as the learners develop mastery over the simple aspects of the skill, and be adjusted to the capability of the learner to understand them—but most of these generalizations are without any scientific support. Although these statements could be true, there is danger in accepting them uncritically, and evidence for such statements should be sought before these conclusions are accepted as guides for behavior in the classroom.

There is little doubt that *some* instruction is necessary for performance of any motor task. Imagine the bewilderment of an individual who is placed before a complex-looking piece of laboratory apparatus and told simply to "begin." Clearly, the performer needs to have some instruction as to what he is to do, how he is to proceed in doing it, and how the performance is scored or evaluated so that he can attempt to maximize some aspect of his responses. Beyond this initial instruction, however, there is the question of how to actually perform the task in terms of the manner of grasping the apparatus, moving it, and so on; evidence from Davies (1945), for example, indicates clearly that such instructions are important in learning archery. There is little evidence to be found, however, on the *nature* of such instructions in terms of their complexity or how complexity should be varied as the skill level increases.

Verbal Pretraining
Other types of information that can be given to learners before practice fall under the heading of *verbal pretraining*, that is, instructions about, or practice with, the stimuli that will be

encountered in actual practice. For example, the regularities of events that occur as the learner is performing the task are important, and he can be asked to learn the sequence of events in the hope that he will transfer this learning to the sequence of events that actually occurs in practice. For example, Adams and Creamer (1962) had subjects learn to follow a sine wave (a regular, smooth, alternating wave form) by moving a hand control. When subjects were allowed to simply watch the wave before trying to track it, responding to the changes in direction with vocal responses, they subsequently performed the tracking task more accurately than did subjects who were not allowed this prepractice activity. Also, Trumbo, Ulrich, and Noble (1965) used a "step-tracking" task (where the track moved in discrete steps) in which the order of steps was regular (e.g., position 1, 3, 5, 2, 4, 6, presented repeatedly), with the subject following the steps with a hand control. When subjects learned the numerical order of the steps before actual practice, they performed the task with considerably greater accuracy than did subjects without this pretraining.

That various instructions about the regularities of the task are important to initial performance is in keeping with the ideas presented earlier concerning the stages of learning (Chapter 4). If it is true that the initial stages of practice are controlled largely by verbal/cognitive activities, it is not surprising that practice on the verbal components of the task have such strong effects on initial performance. By this same argument, however, later in practice, when the verbal components of the task have been learned and the subject is learning the more "motor" aspects of the task, such instructions should be rather ineffective in providing improved learning. In general, then, it would seem that the effects of verbal pretraining and instructions should be important in early practice and should become less important as the task becomes well learned, but there is little research evidence to support this supposition.

Knowledge of Mechanical Principles
Many physical educators have held the belief for some time that a knowledge of the mechanical principles that underlie either (1) the apparatus and its functioning or (2) the move-

ments of the performer's own limbs and body mass, or both, are important to the learning of motor tasks. Perhaps knowledge of these principles could help the learner to choose more appropriate movements and strategies in order to deal with the physical objects in the environment. There is some support for this contention from Mohr and Barrett (1962), who studied the learning of swimming strokes. They provided instructions about the mechanics of swimming, in terms of the laws that governed the propulsive and resistive forces in water, and found that individuals who had such instruction performed better in the swimming tests than did individuals without such instruction. Similar results were found earlier by Broer (1958) with various ball games.

There is not a great deal of evidence about the usefulness of a knowledge of mechanical principles in learning other skills, or about its effectiveness at various points in the learning process. However, on the basis of what is known about the shift in the structure of abilities from cognitive to motor as practice continues, one might predict that the influence of mechanical knowledge might diminish as the task becomes well learned. Once the basic strategies and movement methods for performing the task are established in early learning, further elaboration of mechanical principles should be largely ineffective.

VARIABLES ACTING DURING PRACTICE
Massed Versus Distributed Practice

One of the fundamental variables defining the make-up of the practice session is the scheduling of practice and rest pauses. When practice trials are separated by large amounts of rest, with the rest between trials being as long as or longer than the time in the trial itself, the practice session is said to be "distributed"; when the amount of rest is shorter than the practice, the session is said to be "massed." In practical applications as well as in the laboratory, the schedule of the practice session is set in advance by the instructor or experimenter, and the effect of the degree of massing on the learning of motor tasks is of critical importance in making these decisions. Another consideration is that for a given amount of *practice time* decreasing the rest pauses between trials will increase the number of trials that can be conducted in that period, and the number of trials is known to be important to learning. Therefore, the possible negative effect of the degree of massing combined with the possible positive effects of providing more practice trials need to be taken into consideration in structuring practice.

Continuous tasks. During the 1930s and 1940s, a great deal of data collected indicated that massed practice of continuous motor tasks provided performance inferior to that obtained by distributed practice. A typical example comes from Kimble (1949), who studied the effect of different degrees of massing on the performance of the alphabet-printing task, a task in which the subject tried to print the letters of the alphabet upside-down and backward as quickly as possible. Kimble allowed the subjects to have either 0, 5, 10, 15, or 30 sec rest between 30-sec practice trials, depending on the group to which the subject was assigned, and all subjects had 21 practice trials. With increased massing (decreased intertrial rest) the subjects performed more poorly, and the differences became greater as practice trials progressed. One conclusion was that massing had interfered with the *learning* of the motor task, and many textbooks dealing with motor skills and educational psychology have interpreted these data to mean that massed practice is inferior to distributed practice for learning.

However this conclusion may not be correct because it needs to be shown (as discussed in Chapter 3) that the decrements in performance caused by massing are due to decrements in *learning*. There are two possible sources of the decrement in Kimble's data. One is that the subjects could have learned less because practice was massed, but the other is that massing caused a decrement in *performance* (because the subjects were tired, bored, etc.) and that there was no learning decrement at all; of course, both could be operating. This problem was solved for the first time by Adams and Reynolds (1954), who studied massed and distributed practice on the pursuit rotor. They used five groups of subjects. One group had distributed practice throughout. All of the other groups had some massed practice followed by a 5-min rest and then distributed practice (the "transfer design" mentioned in Chapter 3), with the groups having either 5, 10, 15, or 20 massed trials before switching. The results are shown in Fig. 6.1. There was a great depression in performance while the subjects were undergoing massed practice, but once they were allowed to rest and were shifted to the distributed conditions, the decrement nearly disappeared; in fact, the decrement was gone by the third practice trial after the switch in every case. The conclusion from this study must be that massed practice has large and severe depressing effects on *performance* but that it has minimal effects on *learning* of the motor task. Thus, unraveling the performance versus learning effects of the massing variable revealed it to be relatively unimportant for *learning*, contradicting the conclusions from the earlier literature, which did not

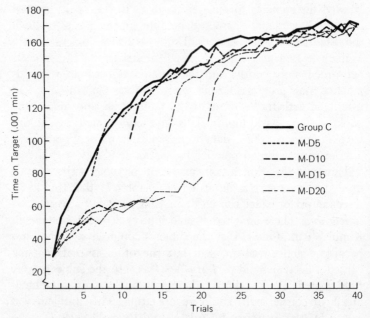

Fig. 6.1 Performance curves for group C with distributed practice throughout and for four experimental groups with massed practice followed by a shift to distributed practice after rest. (From Adams and Reynolds, 1954.)

use a transfer design to separate these two sources of decrement. This conclusion has been supported many times by investigators since this original study with essentially similar results: Massing does not affect the amount of learning in motor tasks. (See, e.g., Stelmach, 1969; Whitley, 1970.)

This conclusion is sometimes difficult for teachers of motor skills to accept. It is curious that learners are able to practice motor tasks under apparently ineffective practice conditions such as heavy massing and still learn as much as individuals who practice under seemingly more "ideal" conditions; however, there can be little doubt from the large body of evidence collected on this topic so far that they can. An important conclusion from the literature on massing is that the level of performance while the subject is learning the task may not reflect the amount that he is learning; this conclusion has important practical implications for the teacher, who has usually been taught that practice must be under ideal conditions for learning to be most efficient.

There are at least a few cases where the above generalization may not hold, however. If the individual is involved in a task in which there is a strong element of danger (such as gymnastics or diving), practice conditions that lead to low-level performances (such as massing) may be undesirable because of the risk of the learner injuring himself. Under such conditions distributed practice would seem more desirable. In addition, if the task is such that a great deal of physical work is required to perform it, providing massed practice may have the effect of not allowing fatigue from the task to dissipate, and the massed practice could be inferior to distributed because of the effects of fatigue on learning the task. Caplan (1970) used two conditions of massing (0 or 30 sec rest with 15-sec trials) on the Bachman ladder task. The learners had to climb a novel, free-standing ladder until they lost balance, whereupon they resumed climbing, the score being the total of the rungs climbed over the 15-sec trial. The Bachman ladder task requires considerable effort to perform well, and subjects typically display signs of fatigue after a few trials of practice. Caplan found that massed practice on the Bachman ladder produced less learning than did distributed, supporting the notion that massed practice with a task of high work load may produce decrements in learning. Therefore, while the generalization that massing is not a learning variable may hold for some tasks, situations in which fear is present, or in which the work load for the task is high, may result in massing being a learning variable.

Discrete tasks. The effect of massing on performance and learning is somewhat different for discrete tasks, however. For example, Carron (1967) varied the intertrial interval on a peg-turn task, in which the subject had to take his finger off a key, reach forward and turn over a peg in a small hole, and return to the original key. The intertrial intervals varied from 7 sec to a nearly incredible 0.30 sec for the various groups. He found that massing had little or no effect in performing the task and no effect on learning the task. The practice time for a discrete task such as throwing a ball is very short for each trial, and it is apparently difficult for massing to cause a build-up of fatigue or boredom in so short a period. All evidence seems to say that massing is not important for either learning or performance with discrete tasks.

How should one structure the learning session with regard to the degree of massing so that learning is maximized? If we have a practice period of, say, 20 min in which to teach a motor skill to students, the evidence seems to say that we should provide as many practice trials as we can in that period —that is, greatly mass the practice—to maximize learning. Even if there might be some slight negative learning effect of the massing, this will be counteracted by the fact that many more practice trials can be given in that period, and the number of practice trials is recognized as a strong determiner of the amount of learning. Except for tasks in which there is a danger of injury, or in which there is a great work load associated with performance, it would seem best to greatly mass practice. Even though this conclusion may be hard for the teacher to accept, the evidence seems clear in support of it.

Physical Fatigue
We all know from our own experiences that when we are greatly fatigued, our skilled performances become impaired. For

this reason, most teachers of skills have avoided attempting to teach motor skills when fatigue was present, thinking that fatigue would cause inappropriate movements that would impair the learning. This conclusion, based as it was on the assumption that fatigue ought to be "bad" for learning, was not really examined scientifically until the early 1960s.

Following initial work on fatigue and learning by Alderman (1965), a number of researchers attempted to provide laboratory conditions in which subjects were fatigued before initial practice on the task, and then performed fatiguing activities between each pair of practice trials to ensure that the level of fatigue was approximately maintained during subsequent practice. For example, Godwin and Schmidt (1971) used women subjects on the sigma task, in which subjects grasped an arm with attached handle, rotated the arm clockwise one revolution until it hit a stop, reversed the direction to rotate counterclockwise for one revolution, and then released the handle and moved 11 inches to knock over a barrier. The score was the time required to complete the designated sigma-shaped (σ) movement. One group of subjects practiced under nonfatigued conditions (group NF), while the other group (group F) cranked an arm ergometer (a friction device to produce fatigue in the right arm) for 2 min. before the first trial. They cranked the ergometer again during each inter-trial interval for 20 trials. All subjects returned to the laboratory three days later for practice (10 trials) under nonfatigued conditions. These results are shown in Fig. 6.2. Fatigue caused large day 1 decrements in performance, as evidenced by the slower movement times for group F. However, on day 2 the decrement present on day 1 decreased somewhat, indicating that all of the day 1 decrement was not due to the effects of fatigue on *learning* of the task, with most being due to the temporary effects on performance. In fact, the differences decreased over the 10 trials on day 2, so that there were only small differences in learning at the end of the second practice period. Conclusions were that fatigue was a large performance variable and a relatively smaller learning variable. Other studies have shown similar results.

What is the practical implication of these findings? While it is true that fatigue did produce decrements in learning, the

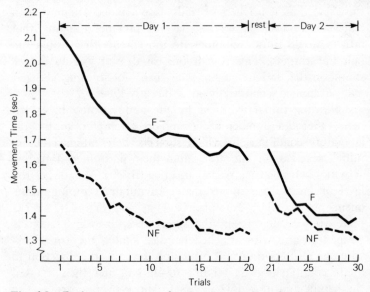

Fig. 6.2 Performance curves for the sigma task under fatigued (F) and nonfatigued (NF) conditions on day 1 and under nonfatigued conditions on day 2. (From Godwin and Schmidt, 1971.)

decrements were very small. Further, fatigue in group F was intentionally maintained at a high level so that the effects, if any, on learning might more easily be seen. Investigators who did not produce such high levels of fatigue, or who did not maintain these levels, have failed to produce fatigue effects on learning. On the contrary, fatigue levels in a class situation would not be intentionally maintained during learning, and since recovery from any existing fatigue is very rapid, fatigue in the teaching situation would seem not to be a serious problem. Nevertheless, fatigue must be classed as both a learning *and* a performance variable.

Specificity of Learning Hypothesis
The specificity of learning hypothesis, borrowed from exercise physiology, says that the practice conditions should agree as closely as possible with the conditions under which the task is to be finally performed. For example, one typically plays hand-

ball in a somewhat fatigued state, and the specificity of learning view would argue that one should practice handball shots while in the same state of fatigue, so that the practice will be most effective for game-type performances.

A recent study by Barnett, Ross, Schmidt, and Todd (1973) tested this view. They asked whether the fatigue state during practice should simulate the actual criterion performance conditions (as in the handball example) in order that practice be most effective. They used the sigma task and provided practice on day 1 under either fatigued (F) or nonfatigued (NF) conditions, as Godwin and Schmidt had. These two groups were then divided again to form four groups for day 2 practice, with the groups having either the same conditions of practice as on the first day (e.g., F-F or NF-NF) or different conditions (e.g., F-NF and NF-F). The day 2 results are shown in Fig. 6.3. When the criterion (day 2) performance was under rested conditions (groups F-NF and NF-NF),

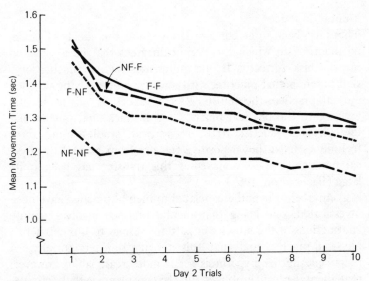

Fig. 6.3 Day 2 performance curves for the sigma task for the four combinations of day 1 and day 2 practice conditions. (From Barnett, Ross, Schmidt, and Todd, 1973.)

day 1 practice under the same conditions (i.e., rested) provided more learning than day 1 practice under fatigued
conditions; this agreed with the Godwin-Schmidt experiment.
However, when the criterion (day 2) task was performed
under fatigued conditions it made little difference whether the
day 1 practice was under fatigued or nonfatigued conditions;
in fact, group NF-F appeared to be slightly faster than group
F-F, indicating that there was some tendency for the practice
under the nonfatigued conditions to be the best for *both* the
day 2 fatigued and nonfatigued task. This clearly contradicts
the specificity of learning hypothesis, since the fatigued task on
day 2 should have been more efficiently learned under
fatigued conditions on day 1. It would appear from these data,
therefore, that practice under the most "ideal" conditions
might be best for learning, regardless of the conditions under
which the task is to be finally performed. This conclusion
should be taken cautiously, however, as it is based on only one
study, and further work must be done before it can be accepted
as law.

Mental Practice

There has been some concern lately about the effects of "mental practice" in which the learner imagines that he is performing the task correctly. If one group uses mental practice of a
skill before actual practice, with another group having no such
mental practice, the transfer (see Chapter 5) of the mental
practice to the physical practice can be measured on the first
few physical practice trials. In general, studies using these
techniques have shown positive transfer from mental to physical practice, and in some cases this transfer has been quite
large (Richardson, 1967).

A number of hypotheses related to mental practice have been
investigated, one being that mental practice involves minute
contractions of the muscles in patterns similar to those in actual
physical practice and that this activity transfers to physical
practice. Another hypothesis seem more reasonable, however:
that mental practice utilizes the strategies and verbal activities
that are known to be a part of the task in the early stages. By
practicing mentally, one can establish appropriate strategies,

review the efforts on previous trials, think about possible errors and how to correct them, and so on; it is little wonder that this kind of activity is beneficial to early performance. But as practice continues, mental practice is less effective and eventually has no effect at advanced levels.

CHAPTER 7

KNOWLEDGE OF RESULTS AND FEEDBACK

The material that follows could have been easily included in the previous chapter since it concerns information the learner receives while he is practicing a motor skill, some of which is under the control of the experimenter or teacher. However, because feedback and knowledge of results are of such great importance to motor learning and performance, they are treated separately here.

FEEDBACK VERSUS KNOWLEDGE OF RESULTS

It is clear that individuals are able to obtain a great deal of information about their performances in a number of ways, and it is convenient to divide them according to the source of information. One class of information is termed *knowledge of results* (KR) and is usually defined as the information provided *by the experimenter* concerning the subject's success. In a positioning task the experimenter might say after a trial "long 12," meaning that the subject moved 12 units too far; alternatively, he could simply say "long," meaning that he moved too far, or he could say "correct" if the movement was within set limits of correctness. Thus KR can have nearly any degree of exactness; it usually refers to how the subject did in terms of the score he is trying to achieve and comes *artificially* from the experimenter or teacher.

Just because the experimenter or teacher does not provide KR on a particular trial does not mean that the subject has received no information about his performance. There are other sources of information, which are termed *feedback*. Of course, the individual can *see* that the ball went through the basket and can *hear* that he struck the ball with the bat, and these sources of information provide additional cues as to the success in the motor response. In addition to visual and auditory information, the learner often receives feedback about the *amount of force* produced via the receptors in the tendons, the *locations of the limbs* via the receptors in the joints, the *pressure exerted* via the touch receptors in the skin, and the *location of the body in space* (upside-down versus right-side-up, accelerating versus decelerating, etc.) via the vestibular apparatus in the inner ear. These sources of information provide a rich source of stimuli to inform the learner of his performance in the task.

THE LAWS OF KR

No Learning Without KR

The most important findings from the KR literature concern whether learning can occur at all without feedback information. (See Bilodeau, 1969.) Bilodeau, Bilodeau, and Schumsky (1959) were not the first to study this question, but their study is reported here because it is modern and makes the point well. They used a positioning task in which learners had 20 trials to learn to make a movement of a given length while blindfolded.

The learners had no direct visual information concerning their correctness, and kinesthetic information was not adequate since they had never experienced the "feel" of the correct response; thus the only information as to error had to come from the experimenter in the form of KR. One group received KR after every practice trial, and one group received no KR at all; the plot of absolute errors is shown in Fig. 7.1. As can be seen, there was no improvement in performance without KR, while the group with KR showed considerable improvement over the 20 trials. Further, when the no-KR subjects were given KR after the twentieth trial, they showed nearly the same improvements that the KR group did, indicating that there was no transfer from the no-KR conditions. Clearly, these data show that learning cannot occur without some information about *errors* (the discrepancy between the actual and correct response).

An exception to this principle is the finding that learners without KR tend to produce responses that are more and more

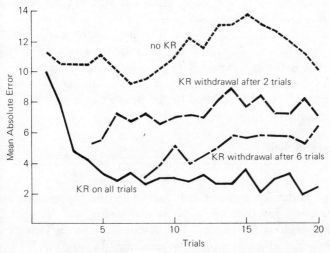

Fig. 7.1 Performance curves on a linear positioning task for groups with and without KR and for groups with KR withdrawn after either two or six trials. (From Bilodeau, Bilodeau, and Schumsky, 1959.)

consistent (but incorrect); that is, they tend to do the same thing to a greater extent as practice continues. This is a kind of learning, to be sure, but the important question is whether the individual can produce responses without KR that are more and more *correct* in terms of the response that is defined by the experimenter (or teacher) as correct. The answer to this question seems to be clearly no.

Frequency of KR

If KR is necessary for learning, how often should it be administered? Is it necessary, for example, to provide KR after every trial, or can the performer be given error information after a number of responses? This question concerns the issue of *absolute frequency* of KR (the total number of KRs given in a trial sequence) versus *relative frequency* of KR (the proportion of trials on which KR is provided). Bilodeau and Bilodeau (1958a) studied four groups using a blindfolded linear positioning task, providing KR after every trial, or after every third, fourth, or tenth trial. Performance improved only on those trials immediately following the presentation of KR, and error remained about the same when KR was not provided. They then plotted the error scores for only those responses that followed the presentation of KR. The performances of these responses were nearly identical for the various groups, indicating that it is the *number* of KRs provided in the learning sequence (absolute frequency) that determines learning and that the relative frequency (related to the number of no-KR trials between KR trials) is unimportant for learning.

Accuracy of KR

How accurate must this error information be? For example, as a limit, one could simply provide KR in terms of "right" or "wrong" as defined by some criterion set by the experimenter. Or one could say that the response was wrong, and in what direction, such as "too long." The exactness of the KR could be increased further by telling the individual by how much he was wrong and in what direction, such as "long 12"; or this information could be further refined by increasing the precision of the KR, such as "long 12.5" or "long 12.56."

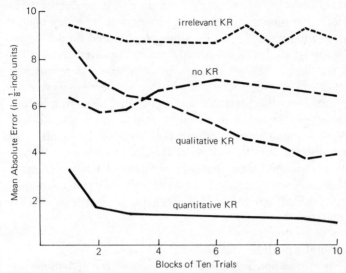

Fig. 7.2 Performance curves on a line-drawing task for groups with no KR, irrelevant KR, qualitative KR, or quantitative KR. (From Trowbridge and Cason, 1932.)

A rather old, but nevertheless informative, study on the precision of KR was done by Trowbridge and Cason (1932). The learner's task was to draw a 3-inch line while blindfolded, with KR in terms of line length provided in a number of ways. One group was given no KR, while another group was given a nonsense syllable after each trial. Another group was given "qualitative KR"; that is, the experimenter said either "right" or "wrong." One final group was given "quantitative KR"; that is, the experimenter said "plus 1" if the response was ⅛ inch too long, "minus 3" if the movement was ⅜ inch too short, and so on. The curves are shown in Fig. 7.2, and it can be seen that there was no learning with either nonsense syllables or no KR. With KR, however, there was considerable improvement, the greatest improvement being with "quantitative KR."

Beyond the improvement in learning from saying "right" or "wrong" to providing quantitative information, there is little further gain in learning or performance when the accuracy of error information is increased. Bilodeau and Rosenbach (1953) showed that numerically rounding the error score to the nearest unit, or multiple of 5, 10, . . ., 50 units, produced no differences in learning, except that in early practice greater accuracy of KR was best. Although it is possible that the experimenter or teacher can provide *too much* accuracy in the KR, there is no evidence from the literature to support this idea. In addition, information about the direction of error alone is more beneficial for learning than is information about the magnitude of error alone, and both sources of information are most beneficial. In summary, then, increased accuracy of KR with respect to direction and magnitude of error leads to greater learning, but the added benefit becomes smaller and smaller as the KR accuracy increases.

Temporal Location of KR

The next question is *when* after a response the KR should be given. Here the learner makes a response, receives KR about that response, makes the next response, receives KR about it, and so on. Fig. 7.3 shows this schematically. The interval from a given response to the next response is termed the *interresponse interval*, and this interval can be divided into two components. The first component is the interval from the response until KR for that response; it is termed *KR delay* because it reflects the amount of time that KR is delayed from the response it describes. The second interval is the *post-KR delay*; it is the time from KR until the next response is performed. Thus the sum of KR delay and post-KR delay is equal to the interresponse interval.

During the KR delay interval, the learner is presumably holding in store important aspects of the response he has just made and is awaiting the information from the experimenter

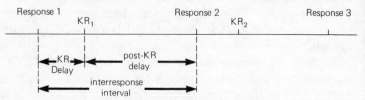

Fig. 7.3 Diagram of events in a learning trial.

concerning the correctness of those movements. During the post-KR delay interval, the learner has received the error information and is evaluating it and formulating a new response for the next trial. Thus, the processes that are occurring during these two intervals are thought to be quite different, and the effects of the various intervals on learning the motor task have been studied to obtain information about those processes.

KR delay interval. Motor behavior researchers expected to find that increasing the KR delay interval would reduce the rate of learning or the level of performance because the analogous effect is so strong in animals. Consider attempting to train a laboratory rat to press a bar when a buzzer sounds and "rewarding" this response by presenting food when it is completed. If one increases the delay from the response until the reward, the learning of the response will be retarded drastically. Since many researchers believed that KR acted as a "reward" for appropriate responses in human beings, it was expected that delay of the KR reward would cause decrements in learning of motor skills. This effect never materialized, as we shall see.

There have been quite a few studies done on the KR delay interval, but one by Boulter (1964) illustrates the point quite well. The task was to make a manual 3-inch movement, and KR was given after every trial in terms of the direction and extent of error. One group had immediate KR, and the other had a KR delay of 20 sec. There were 40 trials, a 2-min rest, and then 8 more trials. KR delay had no effect on learning. Others have produced similar findings, but Bilodeau and Bilodeau (1958b) have provided the most convincing case. They conducted five experiments, each varying KR delay with delays *up to one week*, and failed to show that KR delay has any effect on the acquisition of motor skills. To date, there is no evidence that KR delay is a factor in the acquisition of skills.

What does this mean about the status of KR versus the food reward in animal studies? Since the delay of reward variable has such large detrimental effects in animals, and since KR delay has no effect in human beings, this would lead one to suspect that KR is not "rewarding" as food is for the rat. Most researchers now believe that KR works by being *informative*, providing the learner with information about how he has just responded. (For a review of the information versus reward effects of KR, see Locke, Cartledge, & Koeppel, 1968.) From a practical point of view, the teacher probably does not need to worry about providing "instant information" about the learner's performance, as this information can be delayed considerably without reducing learning, a conclusion that is contrary to usual textbook information. (See, e.g., Deese, 1967, p. 213.)

However, there is one important exception to this conclusion: those situations where KR is delayed for more than the length of the interresponse interval. For example, if I perform the first trial, then the second trial, and *then* I receive KR from the first trial, I have another response coming between a given trial and its KR. This is symbolized in Fig. 7.4, and has been termed the *trials delay* technique. Using a linear positioning task, Bilodeau (1956) varied the number of responses between a given response and the KR that referred to it, using values of 0 (no intervening responses), 1, 2, 3, 4, and 5 trials delay. She found that increased trials delay interfered drastically with the learning of the task, with the greater the trials delay the slower the learning. This is one clear situation where the delay of KR is important to the motor skills teacher. For those cases where the student performs a number of responses, and then is given KR about some aspect of the first of the responses in the series, the KR is likely to be nearly totally ineffective. As a rule, then, one should not worry about the simple delay of KR, provided that additional responses do not come between the response and its KR.

Post-KR delay interval. During the post-KR delay interval the learner presumably "processes" the KR information and

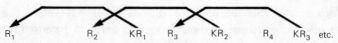

Fig. 7.4 Diagram of the "trials delay" procedure where the trials delay is one.

decides what to do on the next trial. Such decisions might include new strategies, changes in the existing response to correct error, and forming new hypotheses about the nature of the motor problem being solved. Weinberg, Guy, and Tupper (1964), using a positioning task, found that post-KR intervals of 5, 10, and 20 sec produced about the same level of learning but that a post-KR delay of only 1 sec produced poorer learning than the longer intervals. Apparently, some minimal time must be available to process KR information in simple motor tasks, and 1 sec was probably not sufficient. If this is true, shortening the post-KR delay intervals should have larger negative effects as the task becomes more complex because of the greater amount of KR information to be processed; but there are no motor skills data that provide us with this answer. However, data from Bourne and Bunderson (1963), with a concept formation task (in which the learner made successive guesses about the "rule" or concept that governed the members of a complex visual display), showed that shortening the post-KR interval had rather severe effects on learning the concept. Therefore, it would appear that the post-KR interval provides a time for processing KR information and that restricting the time drastically will interfere with learning; also the simpler the motor task, the more the post-KR delay can probably be shortened without disturbing learning.

KR Withdrawal

In most tasks in the everyday world, KR may be provided while the learner is in the initial stages of practice, but eventually he must perform the task on his own without KR. Since Bilodeau et al. (1959) have shown that *some* error information must be provided in order that individuals continue to perform adequately, the learner must shift the source of his error information from the experimenter-generated KR to some form of self-generated error information. Somehow, the individual must be able to use the feedback information from eyes, ears, joints, and so on, he receives on every practice trial to produce *for himself* an error score that closely describes his actual performance. The process of generating one's own error signal has been termed *subjective reinforcement*.

Subjective reinforcement. While it might seem clear that individuals are able to learn to provide subjective reinforcement, evidence supporting this view has not been all that strong until recently. Using a motor task in which the subject had to move a slide along a trackway a distance of 9 inches in exactly 150 msec, Schmidt and White (1972) asked subjects to guess their movement times before the experimenter provided KR as to the actual time (see Chapter 4). At the end of 170 trials, the subjects were remarkably good at guessing their times, the mean difference between what they guessed and what they actually did being only 7 msec. Thus, this evidence indicates that subjects can develop, over the course of practice with KR, the capability to detect accurately their own errors.

Given an accurate self-generated error signal, can subjects use this error information to maintain performance or to *learn* when KR is withdrawn? Schmidt and White found that when KR was withdrawn very early in practice (after the second trial) performance deteriorated considerably for the next 15 trials, indicating that subjective reinforcement was not sufficiently strong to maintain performance. However, when KR was withdrawn after either 20 trials or 150 trials, performance was maintained, and there was even a suggestion that the learning in the task had continued. This indicates that an error detection mechanism was developed over practice that could be substituted effectively for KR.

Error detection mechanism. A number of theories attempt to explain how the error detection mechanism operates and how it is developed; many of them depend on the use of feedback from the various receptors (e.g., eyes, ears, joints, muscles). A theory by Adams (1971) assumes that over the course of practice with KR the learner receives on each trial a representation of how the response felt, looked, and sounded. As the learner gains proficiency in the task, each of these representations form a composite representation of the feedback qualities of the *correct* response; Adams has termed this the *perceptual trace.* Then, when KR is withdrawn, the individual can compare the feedback from the present response with the perceptual trace, and this comparison provides the basis for the error detection mechanism. This perceptual trace should develop more accurately if the movements and the apparatus provide abundant feedback information (e.g., via vision, audition, kinesthetic receptors). Schmidt and Wrisberg (1973) tested this prediction from the Adams theory by having subjects try to make a 20-inch movement of a slide in exactly 200 msec, and either provided "standard" feedback (with vision and audition) or "limited" feedback (no vision or audition). The results are shown in Fig. 7.5. When KR was withdrawn, performance deteriorated, but notice how much less the group with standard feedback deteriorated as compared with the limited group. The interpretation was that the increased feedback from vision and audition caused the subjects to develop a stronger perceptual trace and to be able to maintain performance through subjective reinforcement more effectively than when feedback was minimal.

As important for motor learning as the topic of subjective reinforcement may be—because eventually all learners must perform the response on their own—it is surprising that so

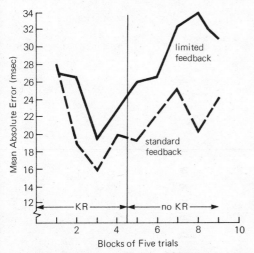

Fig. 7.5 Error in making a 200-msec movement before and after withdrawal of KR and as a function of visual and auditory feedback. (From Schmidt and Wrisberg, 1973.)

little is known about the ways that individuals develop their error detection mechanisms and how the mechanisms operate once they are developed. The area has not been researched very much, but now that there are theories such as Adams' that attempt to explain the subjective reinforcement effect, we should see more research conducted in this area.

CHAPTER 8

THE RETENTION OF MOTOR SKILLS

Up to this point, we have been dealing with the question of how new motor skills are acquired, and now we turn to the question of how well these skills are *retained* over periods of no practice. The typical experimental design for the study of retention provides some practice for individuals to learn a motor task; a period of no practice (called the "retention interval"), during which the individuals are not allowed to perform the motor task; and, finally, "recall trials" of the task. If the performance on the recall trials is in some way less proficient than was the performance of the original learning trials, the subjects are said to have undergone a "retention loss."

RETENTION AND FORGETTING
Forgetting as a Loss of Habit

Retention losses are often considered to be equivalent to forgetting, but a distinction between these concepts is usually made. Just as improvements with practice were assumed to be the result of gains in *habit strength* (learning), forgetting is seen to be the *loss* in habit strength over the retention interval, and it is this habit loss that is responsible for the retention loss. However, just as not all gains in performance are necessarily permanent (and therefore do not represent gains in habit), not all losses in performance are permanent (and therefore are not due to losses in habit). For example, many temporary factors could come into play at the retention test to make performance poor, such as fatigue or boredom, and only if we are sure that these factors are relatively unimportant can we say much about the loss in habit that *is* forgetting.

Absolute and Relative Retention

Consider learners who practice a motor task for 20 trials and then are given a 1-year retention interval, after which practice is resumed. If the level of performance after the retention interval is lower than it was before, we can describe this loss in retention in two ways. *Absolute retention* refers to the level of performance after the retention interval, regardless of where the learners may have left off before the retention interval; it simply states what they did after the retention interval. *Relative retention*, however, describes the *decrement* in retention that has occurred over the retention interval and is usually expressed as the amount of loss divided by the total amount gained (i.e., learned) in the motor task; thus we might say that the relative retention loss was 30 percent, meaning that the drop-off in performance was 30 percent of the total amount of improvement. The importance of these two measures of retention will become evident in a later section.

Areas in the Study of Retention

For convenience, the area of retention can be divided into a number of sections, depending on the nature of the processes thought to cause the decrements. One such cause is thought to be the loss in habit strength for the task ("forgetting"), which can be split into two subdivisions; the first, historically the oldest area, is concerned with the retention of skills that are well learned and is termed *long-term forgetting*, while the second has been concerned with the retention of very poorly learned materials and is termed *short-term forgetting*. The latter part of this chapter is concerned with factors that cause retention losses but that are not thought to involve losses in habit strength, these being the temporary decrements caused by changes in the internal state of the subject.

LONG-TERM FORGETTING
Theories of Forgetting

Trace-decay theory. The oldest and most intuitively satisfying theory of forgetting has been termed the *trace-decay theory*, which states that habit loss occurs spontaneously as a function of no practice on a task. The most important independent variable in the theory is time itself, and the theory states that forgetting *must* occur with the passage of time, with more time causing more habit loss. Opponents of the trace-decay view argue that it is not the mere passage of time, but rather the learning of "interfering" activities, that is responsible for the decrement in performance at the retention test. This argument has lead to the formulation of the *interference theory*, which concentrates on the types of activities that could cause performance decrements.

Interference theory. This theory states that forgetting (habit loss) occurs as a result of "interference" from other learned habits. This interfering activity can occur before the learning of the main task, when it is termed *proactive interference* (PI), or it can occur during the retention interval (between learning and recall of the main task), when it is termed *retroactive interference* (RI), as shown in Fig. 8.1. In studying PI, for example, we concentrate on the control and PI groups at the retention test. If the learning of task B has interfered proactively with the retention of task A, the recall performance of the PI group should be inferior to that of the control group, since the learning of task B before task A was the only way in

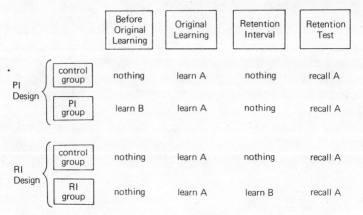

Fig. 8.1 PI-RI design for the experimental study of forgetting.

which these two groups differed. In the RI situation, the effect of learning task B *between* the learning of task A and the recall of A can be evaluated by examining the recall A trials of the control and RI groups. If RI has occurred, at the retention test the control group should show superior recall of A to group RI.

Often students assume that if it can be shown that task B interferes with the recall of task A, the interference theory is "proved" to be true. There is a logical flaw to this conclusion that can be illustrated by the famous "all crows are black" syllogism, as pointed out by Adams (1967, p. 120):

> *A decrement in retention is caused by interference.*
> *Forgetting is a decrement in retention.*
> *Therefore all forgetting is caused by interference.*

The problem is that we may be able to show that so-called interfering activities cause decrements in retention, but we have no evidence that the process that caused the interference decrement is the same process that produces the forgetting seen in everyday activities. Interference decrements are in support of the interference theory of memory, but they do not provide proof of it. (See Chapter 2 for a review of this issue.)

Some Laws of Verbal Forgetting

As most of the research dealing with forgetting has been done with verbal materials, a brief review of the most important findings is useful for understanding the laws of motor memory.

Retroactive interference. There is ample evidence in verbal skills that RI is a powerful determiner of the performance on the retention test. For example, Briggs (1957) had individuals learn a list of paired adjectives, in which a set of stimuli (e.g., red) was paired with a second set of responses (e.g., red-fast). He then presented an "interfering" list, in which the stimuli were the same (e.g., red) but the responses were different (e.g., red-furry). Briggs studied the retention of the original list as a function of both the amount of practice on it and the amount of practice on the interfering list. His results are shown in Fig. 8.2; it is clear that the amount of *decrement* in performance on the original list at the retention test increased with increasing original list practice and increased with increasing practice on the interfering list. The findings agree with the interference theory prediction concerning the worsened recall of one task because of the learning of another task during the retention interval. There is a great deal more evidence for RI in verbal skills, but space does not permit

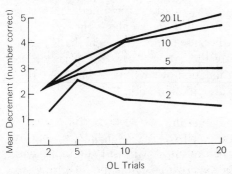

Fig. 8.2 Mean decrement in number of correct verbal paired associates as a function of the number of original practice trials (OL) and the number of interfering practice trials (IL). (From Briggs, 1957.)

treatment of those findings here. Consult Adams (1967, chapter 4) for a review.

Proactive interference. In the early days of the interference theory, the obvious choice for the location of interfering activities was *between* the learning and recall of some task (i.e., RI), and investigators were not concerned with the possibility that learning that occurred before the learning of the main task might cause some forgetting as well. However, Underwood (1957) examined data from a large number of previous investigations that had individuals learning more than one verbal list; he plotted the percentage correct recall as a function of the number of lists that the subject had learned before learning the list in question. The number of such previous lists ranged from one to 20, and it was clear that prior learning was a strong variable for retention, as recall was very good (near 80 percent) when only one list preceded the test list, but was very low (about 20 percent) when as many as 20 lists preceded it, indicating that PI might be a powerful mechanism for forgetting. Perhaps a great deal of the forgetting that occurs in daily life might be due to the PI from all of the learning that has occurred before the learning of the task in question.

In summary, there is a great deal of evidence from the verbal literature that forgetting occurs by a process of interference, but the issue of trace decay versus interference is certainly not settled. A great deal is known about the retention of verbal materials, largely because of the strong emphasis memory research has received over the last few years, the orderly testing of theories, and the formulation of laws. As we shall see, this is not the case in motor skills retention work.

Some Laws of Motor Forgetting

Much of the motor research has been applied (e.g., for military and industrial use) or empirical, without concern for basic laws and theories, the researchers being content to show simply that forgetting did or did not occur. As a result, our knowledge about the causes of motor forgetting is retarded, but a few motor studies do provide some insight into the mechanisms of motor forgetting.

Retroactive interference. The most important work deal-ing with RI in motor skills has come from the University of Iowa, under the direction of Lewis (e.g., Lewis, McAllister, and Adams, 1951). Their study was described in Chapter 5; briefly, they used the three-dimensional Mashburn tracking task and had subjects practice either 10, 30, or 50 trials of the "standard" task, followed by either 10, 20, 30, or 50 trials of the "reversed" task. Decrement in standard task performance as a result of reversed task practice was measured. As was shown in Fig. 5.3 in Chapter 5, there was unmistakable interference from the reversed task to the standard task, and the interference increased both as the number of standard learning trials in-creased and as the number of reversed practice trials increased. Other investigations from the same laboratory have produced similar findings (e.g., McAllister, 1952).[1] Notice that this effect is also present with verbal materials (Fig. 8.2).

As mentioned in Chapter 5, the Iowa studies do not nec-essarily provide evidence for *motor* RI. The writer has argued (e.g., Schmidt, 1971, 1972) that the reversed task may have caused retention decrements because of confusion about "what to do" in response to a given stimulus display and that it may not represent *motor* interference (i.e., "how to do it") at all. In any case, there is clear evidence that some interfering activi-ties can cause decrements in retention, but the implication about the role of interference in the forgetting of motor skills is far from clear.

Proactive interference. In spite of the attention that PI received as a result of Underwood's paper (1957), there has been little work on motor PI. Two studies have been con-ducted, however, but the procedures used have not permitted solid conclusions. For example, Schmidt (1968) attempted to test the interference theory using a task in which the subject had to lift his finger from a key, knock over three barriers in a left-center-right order, and return to the key as quickly as pos-

---

[1] The alert reader will notice that the retroactive interference para-digm is the same as the negative transfer paradigm for transfer research. Thus, RI can be thought of as negative transfer from the learning of a second task during the retention interval.

sible. Four variations of this task were defined in which the location (but not the order) of the barriers was varied. One group learned tasks 1, 2, and 3 before learning task 4, and a control group learned only task 4. If PI was operating to interfere with the retention of task 4, we should expect poorer retention of task 4 for the group that learned tasks 1, 2, and 3 first. However, contrary to the findings in the verbal literature, where "similar" tasks transfer *negatively* to one another, the motor task studied showed a great deal of *positive* transfer (see Fig. 5.2, Chapter 5), and the effect of PI was impossible to determine. It would seem that the operational definitions of "interfering task" and "similar" are considerably different for verbal and motor tasks. This study and an earlier one by Duncan and Underwood (1953) that had similar problems with positive transfer are the only studies that deal with *motor* PI, and little is known about the role of PI in motor skills at present.

Types of tasks. Adams (1967, chapter 4) has discussed evidence that shows that the forgetting of verbal skills is rapid and often nearly complete over rather short retention intervals. In sharp contrast to this rapid verbal retention loss, studies by Fleishman and Parker (1962) using a three-dimensional tracking task, Ryan (1962) using the pursuit rotor, and Meyers (1967) using the Bachman ladder task have all shown almost perfect retention of these skills over retention intervals as long as two years! However, other investigators have found motor skills that were not retained as well, while still others have found rather large retention losses after long retention intervals.

When one examines the wide differences in the degree of retention for these various studies, there appear to be serious contradictions about motor skills retention. However, when the studies are classified in terms of the types of task used, the tasks that show the greatest retention are continuous tracking tasks and those that show the poorest retention are serial manipulative tasks; discrete tasks appear to be approximately intermediate in retention. One possible explanation is that continuous tracking tasks are highly motor, so that the problem for the performer is not what to do, but how to control his movements. On the contrary, serial tasks involve a series of discrete operations (such as throwing switches and levers in a defined order), and learning the order might be more cognitive than are continuous tasks; discrete tasks appear to be intermediate in terms of the motor/cognitive dimension. Therefore, if the idea that the motor components are better retained than the verbal components is true, this might explain the wide differences in retention found in the literature.

Motor versus cognitive components. Not all discrete tasks appear to be cognitive in nature, but those that deal with the pairing of lights and switches, and the like, appear to be. However, there have been a few attempts to study retention with motor discrete tasks. Lersten (1969) used the rho task (a discrete arm movement-speed task involving a circular and a linear component) with retention intervals of 1 year and found that the loss in performance was 79 percent (of the original amount of improvement) for the circular phase and 29 percent for the linear phase. Also, Martin (1970), using a discrete left-arm movement-time task involving knocking over a pair of barriers and returning to a stop switch, found that retention loss was about 50 percent over a retention interval of 4 months, with less loss for shorter retention intervals. Thus, the few studies that have used motor discrete tasks have illustrated that forgetting can be rather large, which does not permit explanation of continuous versus discrete retention in terms of differences in verbal and motor components.

Amounts of learning. Another explanation for differential continuous- versus discrete-task forgetting is that continuous tasks are more *highly learned* than discrete tasks for a given number of trials of practice. Consider the typical 30-sec trial for a continuous task. In that period, there might be a great number of submovements, each of which involves a response to correct an error and each of which presumably develops an increment of habit strength. The discrete task, by comparison, usually involves only one response per trial, with the result that after 10 trials of learning on both tasks, the continuous task might have a great deal more habit strength developed than the discrete task. Since absolute retention depends on the amount of habit strength at the beginning of the retention interval, this could explain why discrete tasks show less absolute retention than continuous tasks. This problem is difficult to solve and would seem to require some method whereby the number of subresponses in continuous tasks could be counted and equated with those for the discrete tasks; this has not been attempted.

What is a "trial"? A third possibility for the continuous-discrete difference in retention concerns the definition of a trial. After the retention interval, a subject is given a trial of the task, and the proficiency on this performance is taken as the measure of the level of retention. With the continuous task, the trial consists of many subresponses, the performance on the continuous trial representing an average proficiency for all the subresponses in that trial. It is therefore possible that the performance on the first subresponse in the trial after the retention interval would show the same degree of performance loss as the first discrete task trial does; however, the subject learns during the trial, so that he is performing very well at the end of 30 sec. Thus, the poor performance on the first subresponse may be "washed out" by the better performance on the latter subresponses. No one has attempted to examine the performance on the first few subresponses in the first trial of the retention test to see if the level of retention might be similar to that shown for discrete tasks.

Other explanations. If the interference theory is true for motor skills forgetting, then discrete tasks, with their somewhat greater dependence on cognitive components, may be interfered with to a greater extent by the vast amount of cognitive learning taking place during the ordinary day. Continuous tasks, being somewhat more motor in nature, may have less motor interference from everyday activities. Another possibility is that continuous tasks are better retained because they are more dependent on feedback (proprioceptive, visual, etc.) for their control than are discrete tasks (Adams, 1967), providing more stimuli to which the responses can become associated during learning. (See Chapter 10.)

There are a great number of hypotheses to explain the difference between the retention of continuous and discrete motor skills, and the issue is still open to question. Unfortunately, these various hypotheses have not been tested, and a full understanding of the long-term retention of motor skills must await the answers.

Motor Versus Verbal Laws

An important approach to understanding skills forgetting involves determining whether or not the laws that describe verbal forgetting are the same as those that describe motor forgetting. If it could be shown that motor and verbal responses follow the same laws, we would be encouraged to believe that they are dependent on the *same processes*; thus the laws generated for verbal materials could be applied to motor skills. On the other hand, if it turns out that motor and verbal skills follow different laws, we will be forced to argue for separate theories of verbal and motor forgetting. The solution to this problem is hampered by the fact that there are not very many laws of motor skills forgetting, thereby permitting only a few comparisons.

One law that has been fairly well established for both types of skills concerns the effect of the degree of learning on the subsequent retention of skills. A related question concerns the effect of "overlearning" on retention, where overlearning is continued practice after subjects have reached some arbitrary level of proficiency and the task is considered "learned." If forgetting is measured by *absolute retention* (the level of proficiency at the retention test), increased overlearning leads to increased proficiency after the retention interval for both motor (Lewis et al., 1951) and verbal (Briggs, 1957) tasks (Schmidt, 1971). If forgetting is estimated by *relative retention* (percentage or *amount lost* over the retention interval), increased learning before the retention interval leads to *decreased* relative retention. That is, learning more before the retention interval leads to greater *losses* over the retention interval for both motor and verbal tasks. (Schmidt, 1971, 1972a.)

A second law of forgetting is that an increased amount of practice on an "interfering task" causes an increased amount of RI; this was shown for both motor (Lewis et al.) and verbal (Briggs) tasks. On the basis of these few laws of forgetting, there is no reason to suspect that motor and verbal forgetting are different processes.

SHORT-TERM FORGETTING

Compared with the long history of research on long-term forgetting, dating back to well before 1900, research on short-term forgetting is very new. Brown (1958) and Peterson and Peterson (1959) presented to subjects a single trigram (e.g., LRT) and prevented them from rehearsing it (i.e., repeating it to themselves) by requiring them to count backward by 3s. Then they asked subjects to recall the trigram after a very short retention interval of up to 18 sec. They found enormous retention losses after this short interval, and these findings led to the idea that this poorly learned information was held in a different "compartment" of memory than was well-learned material. This early work caused a great deal of activity in psychology, with investigators attempting to understand the mechanisms by which the information was lost so quickly.

There was an immediate attempt to determine the cause of this information loss. For example, Hellyer (1962) found that increasing the number of times the trigram was presented (increasing the level of learning) retarded the loss of information. Support for the interference theory was found when Keppel and Underwood (1962) showed that when a series of trigrams was to be presented in sequence the later trigrams were forgotten more easily than the earlier ones, which was evidence for proactive interference.

Short-Term Versus Long-Term Forgetting

It has been tempting to assume that short-term forgetting is different from long-term forgetting, but what is needed to support this assumption is evidence that short-term and long-term forgetting *follow different laws*. Rapid forgetting of poorly learned items could be due to greater long-term habit loss when habit is weak, which does not require assumptions about a different *kind* of forgetting. As a result, researchers have generated evidence that (1) the number of items held in short-term store is only about seven, whereas the number in long-term store is seemingly limitless; (2) meaning is the basis of coding in long-term store, while sound is the basis in short-term store; and (3) well-learned items do not cause interference for poorly learned items. These and other findings have led to the postulation of two storage systems, and some (e.g., Atkinson and Shiffrin, 1971) feel that the short-term store is a kind of "workspace" where information from the environment as well as information from long-term store can be brought together for "processing." It is assumed that information that is poorly learned and stored in short-term store can be "rehearsed" (practiced) and "transferred" to long-term store.

Motor Short-Term Forgetting

During the initial work on motor short-term forgetting, two basic questions were asked: (1) Do verbal and motor short-term forgetting follow the same laws? (2) Is there justification for assuming that short-term and long-term motor forgetting are different systems with different laws? The first motor short-term forgetting study (Adams and Dijkstra, 1966) was patterned after the verbal work, in that the subject made only one response, never rehearsed it, and recalled it after a short retention interval. Blindfolded subjects moved a slide on a trackway until it hit a stop that defined the to-be-remembered position, underwent a retention interval of from 5 to 120 sec, and then attempted to replace the slide in the defined location without the aid of the stop. They found (Fig. 8.3) that the accuracy of positioning was lost rapidly over the short retention intervals. Also, they studied responses with 1, 6, or 15 practice movements as a follow-up to Hellyer's findings for verbal materials and also found that increased practice retarded forgetting.

Interference theory. Since interference had been shown to be such a powerful variable in the verbal work, motor researchers sought to determine the role of interference in motor responses. With respect to proactive inhibition, Ascoli and Schmidt (1969) and Stelmach (1969b) showed (with

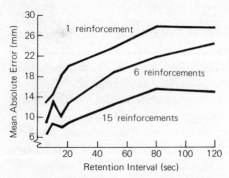

Fig. 8.3 Mean error in a linear positioning task as a function of the length of the retention interval and the number of reinforcements. (From Adams and Dijkstra, 1966.)

positioning responses) that presenting four movements before presenting the movement to be recalled interfered with recall more than with 0 or 2 prior movements. These results conflicted with some later findings by Schmidt and Ascoli (1970), which showed that when 10 positions were presented and recalled in sequence, there was no evidence of poorer recall with later positions, as has been shown in verbal materials (e.g., Keppel and Underwood). Thus it was clear that some kind of proactive interference effects could be shown, but it was not clear that the interference was with the habit for the response or was an artifact of the specific procedures used.

With respect to retroactive interference, however, the picture is much more clear. Stelmach and Walsh (1972) presented a movement to be recalled and then presented additional similar interpolated movements before the actual recall. They found that when the interpolated movements were longer than the criterion movement, the recall movement tended to be too long, and when the interpolated movements were shorter than criterion, it tended to be too short. There are other instances of RI in motor short-term forgetting, and the phenomenon seems to be well established. In summary, there is strong support for RI, with marginal support for PI, giving the interference theory relatively strong status in explaining motor short-term forgetting.

Long-term versus short-term motor forgetting. It was pointed out earlier that long-term and short-term *verbal* forgetting appear to be separate processes governed by separate laws. In contrast, however, the laws that have been generated for short-term motor forgetting appear to hold for long-term forgetting as well. For example, practice tends to make absolute recall of both long-term and short-term items more proficient, the interference theory has some support from both long-term and short-term responses, and so on. Not being able to isolate different long-term and short-term laws would seem to prevent the assumption of two kinds of motor forgetting. However, there have not been very many laws established, and it is possible with new laws there will be sufficient differences to allow the distinction. At this stage, however, a single forgetting process appears to be the most logical choice.

TEMPORARY FACTORS
CAUSING RETENTION LOSS

It was pointed out previously that a retention loss is not necessarily forgetting because temporary factors such as fatigue or boredom could be encountered at the retention test to depress performance. One of the most important of these temporary (nonhabit) factors is the decrement in performance that usually follows a period of no-practice, even when this period is as short as 2 min. Consider Fig. 8.4, which shows the results of practice on a linear positioning task. Subjects received KR after each of 20 trials, with a 10-sec intertrial interval, and then were allowed to rest in a separate room. When they returned to the task after 5 min, subjects showed a decrement in performance that remained for approximately 3 to 4 trials. This decrement in performance has been thought to be caused by the need to "warm up" to the task (psychologically) after the rest and has been termed *warm-up decrement* (WUD). It is a characteristic of nearly every motor task that has been studied in this context and appears after rests as short as 40 sec.

Because WUD is evidenced by reduced proficiency at the retention test, it has been termed the *second facet of forgetting* by Adams (1961). But simply because the decrement "behaves like" forgetting (i.e., habit loss) does not mean that

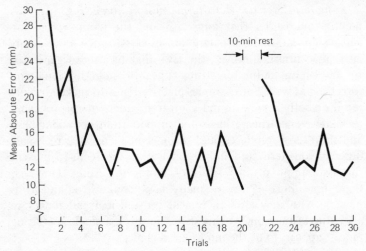

Fig. 8.4 Warm-up decrement evidenced as increased error in a linear positioning task after a 10-min rest. (From Schmidt and Nacson, 1971.)

WUD *is* forgetting; and simply because WUD appears after very short rests and is eliminated quickly with practice—characteristics that seem unlike a forgetting process—does not imply that WUD is a process different from forgetting. What is needed is evidence to show that the laws of WUD are different from the laws of forgetting if the two processes are to have separate status.

Warm-Up Decrement as Forgetting

Some researchers have attempted to rule out the forgetting (habit loss) hypothesis by using "neutral" tasks (whose habit has nothing in common with that for the task to be remembered) in attempts to reduce WUD before the retention test. Following the lead from Irion's work (1948) with WUD in verbal skills, the author and his associates (Nacson and Schmidt, 1971; Schmidt and Nacson, 1971; Schmidt and Wrisberg, 1971) have shown with motor tasks that neutral tasks performed just before recall can reduce subsequent WUD. For example, Schmidt and Wrisberg used a right-hand movement-time task (sigma task) as the main task and allowed subjects to perform a different left-hand movement-time task before recall after a 5-min rest. They found that WUD was less than for a group that simply rested. Since the left-hand and right-hand tasks were assumed not to have habit in common, a forgetting explanation of WUD was rejected. There seems to be considerable verbal and motor evidence that WUD is not simply forgetting.

The Set Hypothesis

Various workers proposed to account for the decrement in terms of one of a number of forms of "set," that is, postural and attentive adjustments that underlie the motor task in question but that are not part of the habit strength for the task. For example, the performer can adjust his posture over the course of practice on the pursuit rotor so that he is in the most efficient position, but when he returns to the task after a rest, the correct posture is lost and must be regained. There have been numerous attempts to test the set hypothesis by specifying neutral (i.e., nonhabit) activities that would reinstate the lost set and reduce WUD after a rest period. In a typical study, Ammons (1951) used the pursuit rotor as the main task and then allowed subjects to rest before having them return for a retention test. During the rest, each subject engaged in "neutral" activities (watched another subject, followed the target with his finger, and the like) to reinstate set. Ammons failed to show that these tasks reduced WUD on the pursuit rotor. Other attempts testing the set hypothesis of WUD have failed as well (see Nacson and Schmidt, 1971, for a review), perhaps because the particular choices for the neutral tasks were inappropriate. However, it is possible that the set hypothesis is wrong, and that WUD is due to some other process than was specified by the set theorists.

The Activity-Set Hypothesis

The activity-set hypothesis also postulates that WUD is due to the loss over rest of a temporary, nonhabit, internal state (termed the *activity set*), but the state is not specific to the particular task. Rather, the activity set is the state of adjustment of each of a number of subsystems that underlie and support the task. For example, the learner needs to adjust his level of excitement (termed *arousal* or *activation*) so that it is compatible with the task, since too much or too little arousal can lead to ineffective performance. Also, he must adjust his attention to various sources of feedback, since some tasks require attention to visual feedback (catching a ball) and other tasks (e.g., wrestling) might require attention to tactual and proprioceptive feedback. The hypothesis says that the performer adjusts all of these systems while he is practicing so that the performance is maximized. In this state, the subject is said to have the appropriate activity set. When he rests he adopts a different pattern of adjustment appropriate for resting, and when he returns to the task he must eliminate the resting pattern and reestablish the pattern appropriate for the motor task. Doing this takes time and he performs poorly until the proper activity set can be reinstated.

One fundamental prediction of the activity-set hypothe-

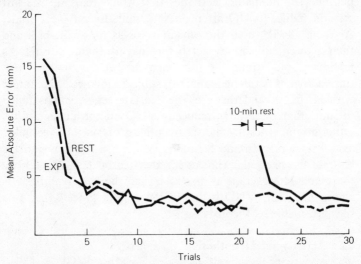

Fig. 8.5 Reduced warm-up decrement in right-hand force-estimation task for group EXP, which practiced a left-hand force-estimation task during the 10-min rest interval. (From Nacson and Schmidt, 1971.)

sis is that practicing any task of the same class (or type) as the main task will reinstate the same activity set and reduce WUD on the main task. Nacson and Schmidt (1971) used a task in which the subject attempted to exert a hand-grip force of exactly 45.4 lb, with KR after each of 20 trials. The subjects then rested for 10 min outside the test room reading magazines, and so on. One group (REST) returned to the force-estimation task directly after resting; another group (EXP) returned to the test room to practice a left-arm force-estimation task (involving flexing the elbow) before practicing the right-hand task. Thus, the activity set for the left and right tasks should be similar, with the left-hand task reinstating the activity set; resuming practice on the right-hand task immediately after the left-hand task should result in little or no WUD relative to the control group, which rested. The results are shown in Fig. 8.5. The WUD was nearly eliminated for group EXP but was large for group REST supporting the predictions from the activity-set hypothesis. Therefore, the evidence presented to date seems to be that WUD is not due to forgetting of the motor responses, but rather is due to the loss over rest of the essential temporary adjustments of the various systems that underlie the motor task.

CHAPTER 9

INDIVIDUAL DIFFERENCES

Up to this point, the major concern of the book has been understanding the mechanisms and processes that underlie motor skills performance and learning. In isolating these processes, the fact that individuals are different from one another in a number of ways has not been considered. In fact, these differences might imply that the processes might be different for different individuals.

The field of psychology (and motor skills as well) can be divided according to two distinct philosophies. The most popular point of view ignores the differences among individuals to concentrate on the similarities; it is termed *experimental* psychology because researchers use experimental methods (see Chapter 2) that emphasize laws that apply to all individuals. The less popular point of view is concerned with the differences among people and is termed *differential* psychology. These two divisions are quite distinct, with individuals in the two "camps" seldom working together.

INDIVIDUAL DIFFERENCES GOALS

An important goal of the differential scientist is to determine to what extent the various laws and principles for motor skills are appropriate for different classifications of individuals (e.g., men versus women; children versus adults) and to modify the laws when necessary. However, the major goal is *prediction*, where individuals' performances on a given task are predicted from knowledge about their performances on other tasks. The prediction of college success (e.g., college grade point average) from college entrance examination scores is a typical example. A major activity of the researcher in individual differences is to develop tests and test batteries that predict certain performances as accurately as possible.

METHODOLOGY

Nearly every study of individual differences involves either (1) the use of "individual difference variables" in pseudo-experiments or (2) the measurement of the relationship between two or more tests with correlations. These are discussed in turn.

Individual Difference Variables

Studies using individual difference variables divide a group into two or more subgroups according to some trait and then assess the "effect" of this trait on some other performance. For example, a group of subjects could be divided according to sex, with males and females being compared on a motor skill to determine the "effect" of sex on skill. This is a pseudo-experiment (see Chapter 2) because the independent variable (sex) is not assigned to the subjects by the experimenter; rather, group membership is dependent on the value of the independent variable. As was pointed out in Chapter 2, if sex differences in performance are found, we are only permitted to conclude that some variable *associated with* sex was responsible for the differences; we have no means for telling precisely what variable caused the differences. Studies of this type are frequent; examples are the effect of sex, race, intelligence, socioeconomic background, and so on, on motor performance.

Correlational Studies

Another very common approach to individual differences involves the use of the correlation coefficient, which measures the degree of relationship (see Chapter 2) between two variables (or tests). We will consider here some of the general characteristics and interpretations of the correlation.

The basic "ingredients" for a correlation are scores from at least two tests measured on a relatively large number of individuals (e.g., heights and weights for 100 students). The computed correlation may vary from -1.00 to $+1.00$, depending on the characteristics of the relationship between the two tests. If the correlation is negative (e.g., -0.80), the relationship is negative, so that large scores on one test tend to be paired with small scores on the other test (e.g., weight and number of chin-ups). A positive sign indicates a positive relationship where large scores on one test are paired with large scores on the other (e.g., height and weight). Therefore, the sign of the correlation indicates only the *direction* of the relationship between the two tests.

The *strength* of the relationship is given by the size of the correlation. Correlations that are close to 1.00 or -1.00 (e.g., -0.95 or $+0.88$) indicate a high degree of association between the two tests, while correlations close to zero (e.g., -0.20 or $+0.15$) indicate weak associations between the two tests. A correlation of zero indicates that there is no relationship between the two tests, while correlations of either 1.00 or —1.00 indicate perfect relationships.

Correlations can be interpreted in a number of ways. If the correlation between two tests is high (e.g., —0.80 or +0.80), the tests are said to measure the same underlying trait. Thus, a high correlation between height and weight indicates that both tests measure the same trait of "body size." On the other hand, when the correlation between two tests is low (close to zero), the tests are said to measure *different* underlying traits. These traits are hypothetical constructs and are frequently termed *abilities* (see Chapter 4).

A frequent use of the correlation is to determine to what extent the two tests are measuring the same underlying ability. For example, if my two tests are reaction time with the left hand and reaction time with the right hand, and I find that the correlation between these two measures is —0.90, then I *infer* that both measures were estimating the same basic *ability* of the individual to react quickly. However, if two tests do not correlate very highly (e.g., +0.05), I infer that they were not measuring the same ability or that the ability that determined the performance of individuals on one test was not the same as that on the other test. Also, a high correlation coefficient between tests A and B does not imply that changes in A *caused* changes in B, since it might be true that a third variable C causes changes in both A and B, resulting in the relationship observed.

MOTOR ABILITIES

We turn now to the concept of underlying motor *abilities*, hypothetical constructs thought to be *innate, relatively stable characteristics of the individual that underlie a certain type of motor response*. If an individual has a weak ability, the responses that depend on that ability will not be proficient, and vice versa; proficient performance is taken as evidence that the underlying abilities are strong.

The concept of an ability should be distinguished from the concept of a *skill*. An ability is thought to be inborn and relatively stable, while a skill is easily modifiable by practice. Also, an ability is thought to be more general than is a skill, with abilities forming the basis of a number of specific skills. For example, we may speak of the ability to move quickly, referring to perhaps a large number of specific movements (skills).

General Motor Ability Hypothesis

The earliest thinking about abilities and motor behavior concerned the idea that all motor skills, ranging from athletics to typing, were based on a singular motor ability, which was termed *general motor ability* (GMA). This view was similar to the ideas prevalent at that time concerning the nature of intelligence; all intellectual skills were thought to be represented by a general intellectual capacity, largely genetically determined and generally unmodifiable by practice and experiences. In the same way, individuals were thought to possess GMA; those who had "good" GMA were able to perform well on nearly any motor task they attempted, and those who had "poor" GMA were destined to fail at nearly every task they tried. The GMA concept was accepted rather uncritically, as it was a satisfying explanation for the apparent performance differences observed on the playing fields. For example, the all-around athlete was thought to have a great deal of GMA, which was responsible for his strong success in many school sports such as baseball and football. By the same reasoning, those individuals who were unsuccessful at nearly every motor skill were thought to have a very poor GMA.

The GMA hypothesis predicts that an individual who possesses a great deal of skill in some motor task (e.g., some sport) should be able to perform well in *any other* motor task he should attempt. To test this view, Henry[1] selected three classifications of athletes (basketball players, rifle team members, and gymnasts) and one group that had never had organized athletics of any kind. He compared these groups on four laboratory apparatus tasks that they had not practiced before: (a) a choice reaction-movement time task, (b) the stabilometer balance task, (c) an apparatus that measured body sway, and

[1] Personal communication (1966) with F. M. Henry, University of California, concerning unpublished data collected in 1950.

(d) a task involving kinesthetic sensitivity. Contrary to the predictions from GMA theory, the specialized athletes supposedly having strong GMA did not outperform the non-athletes, except that the rifle team members displayed less body sway than any other of the groups. Henry concluded that GMA does not exist.

A second line of evidence against the GMA theory comes from an analysis of the correlations among various motor tasks. If GMA exists, then individuals proficient in one task should possess high GMA and should also be proficient in *all* other tasks. This leads to the prediction that motor tasks should show a strong tendency to be associated (or correlated), and the correlation between any two motor tasks should be relatively high. However, numerous studies during the 1950s and 1960s showed that the correlations among motor tasks, even motor tasks that resembled each other strongly, were very low and were sometimes zero.

These two lines of evidence argued strongly against the GMA notion, and it has faded from popularity among motor skills researchers because of lack of evidence supporting it. Unfortunately, the GMA view is still held by many motor skills teachers, and the concept remains with us in the "popular" skills literature. Since there is no support for such a notion, we can only hope that the modern student of motor skills will not adopt such a concept on the say of former coaches and teachers and will evaluate the evidence that is so strongly against the GMA notion.

Henry's Specificity Hypothesis

A view strongly opposed to the GMA ideas was presented formally by Henry (1968). He hypothesized that a very large number of abilities underlie man's motor responding; each of these abilities is responsible for only a very limited number of movements, and even slightly different movements require that different abilities come into play. For example, throwing two different sized balls should involve different motor abilities. With such a large number of abilities proposed, the success in any given performance is largely a matter of the "quality" of the abilities for that particular response. Further, these abilities are thought to be independent of each other. That is, the quality of any one ability for a given person is not dependent on the quality of any other ability. Thus, the individual is seen as having a large number of such *independent* abilities, some of them being "good," some "bad," with most being about average. The "all-around athlete," therefore, is one who, through the predictable and chance factors in genetics, happens to possess a large proportion of the "good" independent abilities.

Because the abilities underlying motor performance are *independent* in Henry's view, so that possessing one good ability does not guarantee the presence of another good one except by chance, we should find that individuals who perform well on one task do not necessarily also perform well in another task. This implies that the correlations between two motor tasks should be close to zero.

An early test of the specificity hypothesis was conducted by Bachman (1961), who studied the correlation between performances on two balancing tasks. One of the tasks used the stabilometer; the subject had to balance on an unstable platform, with the score being the amount of movement (in degrees) during a 30-sec trial. The second task was the Bachman ladder-climb task, in which the subject had to climb a special, free-standing ladder. He began climbing until he toppled over, then began climbing again, until the 30-sec trial was completed; the score was the number of rungs climbed in a trial. All subjects received practice on both tasks, and the scores at the end of the practice period were used as the measure of the ability of the subjects to perform each of the balance tasks. Bachman found that the correlations between the tasks were very low (i.e., less than 0.20) for all age groups tested, with the average correlation for all of the age groups taken together being 0.003. These findings supported the conclusion that there was no underlying ability to balance, and that the two balance tasks were dependent on separate and independent abilities. Numerous other studies have been concerned with this fundamental prediction from the Henry theory. With very few exceptions, the correlations among motor tasks are very low, regardless of the type of task studied, the type and age of subjects used, and so on (e.g., Lotter, 1960). This supports the hypothesis that motor performances are dependent on a large number of *independent* abilities, as Henry has proposed, and rejects strongly the notion of GMA.

Critics of the specificity theory point to the fact that the correlations between motor tasks, admittedly quite low, are almost always positive, while the Henry theory would predict zero correlations on the average, with some negative and some positive by chance. The rather persistent presence of low, positive correlations leads one to the conclusion that motor abilities may not be as independent as the specificity view holds and that there may be abilities common to many motor tasks (e.g., motivation, body configuration). Even if motor abilities are not strictly independent, the correlations among skills are almost uniformly low, permitting poor prediction of success in one motor task on the basis of performance in some other task.

Fleishman's Motor Abilities Hypothesis

The GMA and specificity hypotheses represent extremes in thinking about motor abilities: that all skills are based on *one* ability (GMA), and that every skill has its own ability that underlies it and no other motor skill (specificity). Fleishman's findings (see, e.g., Fleishman, 1965) point to a position between these two views. His method is termed *factor analysis*, in which a large number of subjects (e.g., 300) perform a large number of motor tasks (e.g., 100). The factor analysis technique locates clusters of skills that are correlated (e.g., 0.30) with each other but are correlated 0 with tasks in other clusters; thus out of 100 tasks some 10 or so clusters may be identified. Each of these clusters of tasks (usually termed *factors*) is thought to represent a basic underlying ability, and these abilities are named according to the types of tasks that are in the cluster. For example, one cluster might contain tasks that involve moving a limb rapidly; this cluster might be termed *movement speed*, being evidence for an underlying movement speed ability. Another factor might be termed *static strength* if the majority of the tasks in the cluster involved the exertion of maximal force. Thus, factor analysis allows inferences about the structure of the underlying abilities.

A word of caution is in order about the technique of factor analysis, however. First, it has been criticized because the factors that emerge from the analysis are dependent on the particular tests selected for analysis; if there were no test involving rapid movement, no movement speed factor could emerge. The critics point out that many abilities could be overlooked because the investigator failed to include appropriate tests in the battery. Second, there is a great deal of subjectivity in naming the factors, and two investigators might differ considerably in the names they apply to the same factors. Third, there are a number of different types of factor analysis, and frequently the same data treated with different analyses will produce markedly different results.

Even though the factor analytic work should be viewed with some caution, the results of such studies are useful. A description of some of the abilities outlined in Fleishman's work is presented next.

1. *Control precision.*   Tests that measure this factor require careful positioning of the hands and/or feet, especially when the movement is rapid. It applies to both discrete and continuous performances.

2. *Multilimb coordination.*   This factor is involved in performances where more than one limb is controlled simultaneously. Common examples are driving a car (steering, shift lever, and foot pedals) and swimming.

3. *Response orientation.*   This factor is involved when the individual must choose the correct response from a number of alternatives as quickly as possible (e.g., when a defensive football player moves quickly in the correct direction as the play develops).

4. *Reaction time.*   This factor is concerned with *initiating* a single response as quickly as possible after a stimulus and is measured as the interval from a stimulus until the movement is started. The ability to react quickly is important in a number of activities where stimuli are presented suddenly (e.g., a swimming start).

5. *Speed of arm movement.*   This factor is involved in making rapid, one-directional arm movements when accuracy

is not a requirement. Evidence from Fleishman (1965) and Henry (1961) indicates that the movement speed factor is independent of the reaction time factor, contrary to those who would think of these two factors together as "quickness."

6. *Rate control.* This factor is related to the ability to make movements at a particular rate (not at maximal speed). Since it is related to anticipation of upcoming events, the factor represents "timing," where the problem is to make a particular response at the appropriate time.

7. *Manual dexterity.* This factor involves the movements and control of rather large objects with the arms and hands. It is important in the handling of packages, in assembling large components on assembly lines, and so on.

8. *Finger dexterity.* This is similar to manual dexterity except that movements are smaller, primarily using the hands and fingers to manipulate small implements (e.g., the ability required by a watchmaker).

9. *Arm-hand steadiness.* This factor is involved in tasks in which the limbs must be positioned with speed and strength minimized. This ability represents the amount of limb tremor and is important in tasks such as threading a needle and riflery.

10. *Wrist-finger speed.* This factor represents the speed with which the individual can move the fingers, hand, and wrist. It is sometimes termed *tapping.*

The above list of abilities should not, of course, be seen as a complete representation of human motor abilities. There are many aspects of motor performances that have not been included in factor analytic studies, and future work will undoubtedly reveal new motor abilities and further subdivide the existing ones. Rather, the above list should be seen as evidence supporting Fleishman's idea of a limited number of abilities relating to a rather narrow classification of motor tasks. The evidence from a number of sources seems to support the conclusion that there are a relatively large number of abilities underlying motor performance, that they are relatively independent, and that each encompasses a relatively narrow set of motor behaviors.

MOTOR EDUCABILITY

During the 1930s, motor skills researchers and teachers attempted to develop batteries of tests that would predict the ease with which students could *learn* new motor skills, commonly called tests of *motor educability*. This work closely paralleled the work in psychology concerning intelligence, with the subsequent development of numerous intelligence (IQ) tests; the motor work was aimed at attempting to isolate and define motor IQ. Motor educability was thought of as an ability much like GMA but different in that it supposedly predicted the *learning* of motor skills as opposed to the performance of motor skills. The most famous of these tests was the Iowa Brace test, which utilized a battery of simple movements (e.g., hopping on one foot), each scored on a pass/fail basis.

It was expected that individuals who scored high on motor educability tests would *learn* new motor skills more easily and more quickly than would individuals who scored low on such tests. Gross, Griesel, and Stull (1956) tested this notion with the Iowa Brace test and learning to wrestle and found that learning to wrestle and the Brace test correlated very poorly ($r = 0.20$), contrary to the motor educability notion. A number of other studies have been done using different motor learning tasks with various motor educability tests, and the results are strikingly similar; there is no evidence that motor educability tests predict the ability to learn new motor tasks.

These motor educability findings have two possible interpretations. First, it could be that the early motor educability tests were not particularly well developed and that future tests might better predict the slow and fast motor learner. A second interpretation, however, is that the reason that the motor educability tests did not predict speed of learning was that no such ability to learn exists. This latter hypothesis has been tested recently by investigating the correlation between *learning scores* (i.e., the change from initial to final performance) in one task with learning scores in another task. If an individual learns a great deal in one task, the motor educability view would say that this was a result of having a strong ability to learn, which should show up on a second task in the form of a large learning score; thus the correlation between learning scores on the two tests should be high. Bachman (1961) correlated the learning scores on the Bachman ladder-climb task with learning scores on the stabilometer and found that the correlations were very low, with the average correlation for various age groups being almost 0. Because a number of other studies have reported essentially identical results, we are led to the conclusion that there is no evidence for general ability to learn motor skills. This conclusion should be taken cautiously, however, since it depends on the analysis of habit strength gains by using learning (gain or change) scores, a procedure that is not recommended, as argued earlier (Chapter 3).

PREDICTING PERFORMANCE AND LEARNING

As mentioned earlier, a major emphasis of the work on individual differences in skills is *prediction*. There is a need to be able to predict which individuals will be successful after finishing training in a variety of fields such as pilotry, dentistry, and professional sports; since the training programs for many occupations are expensive and time-consuming, being able to "weed out" those individuals who would not succeed in a program would make the problem somewhat simpler. However, for a number of reasons predicting final performance from pretraining testing batteries has been quite unsuccessful.

Only Fleishman and his colleagues have devoted a continuing research effort toward motor abilities, and our understanding of abilities remains nearly where Fleishman has left off. As a result, our knowledge about the structure of underlying abilities is incomplete, and it is probable that the abilities outlined thus far will be divided into subabilities, and new abilities will be discovered as a result of more inclusive research programs. Those interested in predicting posttraining performance from batteries of tests are having a difficult time, because the abilities (and tests that measure them) are not sufficiently well understood. Thus, the accurate prediction of success in industrial and sports situations must await the more basic work in human motor abilities.

The problem is further complicated by the fact (see Chapter 4) that the pattern of abilities may change markedly as individuals become more proficient in a task. I could, for example, choose employees on the basis of the first few attempts at the task they are to learn to perform, under the assumption that performers proficient initially will be those who will be proficient after learning. While this procedure is often used, it has a number of problems; the correlation between the first few trials of a task and the last few can be very low if there is a great deal of learning, meaning that individuals are ordered (from most to least proficient) differently on the initial test than they are on the final test. Therefore, choosing the "best" individuals on the initial test will not necessarily provide the "best" individuals in the task after learning has occurred. What we need are test batteries that can be administered *before* training that are predictive of performance *after* training. Such batteries, however, are not currently available for most sports or industrial situations.

CHAPTER 10 | THE CONTROL OF MOVEMENT

In this chapter we focus on the individual and his responses after he has practiced a task for some time and his movements are smooth and proficient. The central question is how the individual controls his muscles and limbs so that this skilled performance can be exhibited. If the movement is to be "skilled," the muscles must contract with the proper force, at the proper time, and in the proper order with respect to the other muscles. How the individual organizes himself to accomplish this feat is an exciting question. How does the performer issue the "commands" to the muscles and how are they issued at the proper time? What cues does the individual "pay attention to" as he is performing? Does this information aid performance, and, if so, how does it operate?

There are a number of alternative explanations for how the individual controls his own musculature. One of these is that the subject "programs" his movement in a way analogous to the operation of a computer; thus, the individual has a set of stored programs, each of which dictates the activities of the relevant musculature for a particular movement. Alternatively, we know that the performer receives a great deal of information about the state of his environment and of his own body via feedback, and he could be using the feedback information to somehow determine which muscles are to be contracted next and in what way. To help examine these possibilities, some basic considerations of system control theory are presented next.

CONTROL SYSTEMS
Open-Loop Systems
One simple type of control system is termed an *open-loop* system, and a schematic diagram of such a system is provided in the top part of Fig. 10.1. The system has two separate components: (a) the "executive," which has a decision-making, or command, function, and (b) the "effector," which carries out the commands issued by the executive. To perform a task, the commands are structured by the executive and the instructions are issued to the effector, where they are carried out as ordered. A good example is a traffic signal, which progresses through the sequence of red, amber, and green lights as ordered by preset commands. The system is good because instructions to the effectors can be planned in advance (that is, they can be pre-programmed) and it is very simple. It has the disadvantage of being inflexible in the face of changing situations, for example, the traffic snarl caused by the preprogrammed light sequencing. If the system could somehow be sensitive to moment-to-moment fluctuations in traffic load, it would be more effective.

Closed-Loop Systems
The closed-loop system reduces somewhat the problems of inflexibility in the open-loop system; it is illustrated in the bottom

part of Fig. 10.1. Here the state of the system as affected by the instructed changes in the effector are fed back to the executive, where they are monitored and compared against a *reference value* (the desired state of the system). Subsequent instructions are issued whenever the comparison indicates that the system has not achieved its goal. For example, consider the automatic steering mechanism (a *servomechanism*) in an ocean liner. The automatic pilot (the executive in this case) is set for a certain course. If the electrical feedback from the ship's compass indicates that the ship is not on the desired course, appropriate instructions are issued to the rudder control mechanism (the effector) to turn the ship. New directional information is fed back to the executive, and subsequent corrections are made until the difference between the actual and desired course is zero. Once the ship is on course, deviations that might occur because of sea or wind conditions can be corrected, keeping the ship on course. The use of *feedback*, the determination of an *error* (the difference between the actual and desired direction), and the *correction* of error are characteristic of the closed-loop system.

Theorists interested in human movement recognized early that a great deal of feedback is available in some tasks to guide

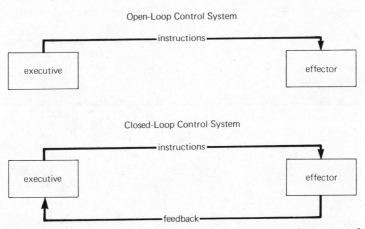

Fig. 10.1 Schematic diagram of open-loop and closed-loop control systems.

performance. Because of the potential for the use of feedback by human beings to control movements it was tempting to visualize the human being as a servomechanism, applying what is known about servo theory to human motor performance. Whether or not we can profitably view man as a closed-loop system is the topic of the next few sections.

DELAYS IN PROCESSING STIMULI
Reaction Time

One of the most important concepts bearing on the servo-mechanism model of the human being concerns the amount of time required for feedback to be "processed" by the executive and for the executive to initiate a response to that feedback. The most fundamental finding concerns the delay in response to an unanticipated signal, a delay termed *reaction time (RT)*. When the subject receives a suddenly presented signal and must react to it by making a response as quickly as possible, the delay in getting the response under way is approximately 0.15 sec under ideal conditions and can be as long as 0.30 sec. This finding indicates simply that individuals cannot react to unanticipated information from the periphery (e.g., eyes, ears) immediately and that some delay in response is nearly always present.

Psychological Refractoriness

A second type of delay is found in the situation in which a first stimulus (S_1) instructs the subject to perform some act (e.g., press a reaction key), and then a second stimulus (S_2) is presented suddenly that instructs the subject to perform a second act (Fig. 10.2). When S_2 is presented unexpectedly the RT to S_2 is somewhat longer than "normal" RT, and the lengthening of RT_2 depends on how close in time S_1 is to S_2. For example, if S_2 follows S_1 by only 0.10 sec (so that S_2 occurs *before* the subject's response begins), the delay in response to S_2 (RT_2) can be as long as 0.50 sec. This delay (called *psychological refractoriness*) has been interpreted (see Welford, 1968) to mean that man is a "single-channel" organism, in which only one signal can be processed at a given

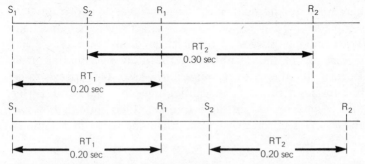

Fig. 10.2 Diagram showing the hypothetical effect of psychological refractoriness as the delay in reaction time to the second of two closely spaced signals.

time. When S_1 appears, the subject is processing it during RT_1 and any signal that appears during RT_1 must have its processing delayed until the single channel has finished processing S_1. When S_2 appears considerably after S_1 (e.g., 0.50 sec after S_1), the single-channel mechanism has already been cleared of S_1, and RT_2 is approximately "normal." This additional limitation implies that if a second signal (for example, a signal to change a movement or to perform some new movement) appears close to the first, there can be a very long delay in responding to it.

FEEDBACK DELAYS AND MOVEMENT CONTROL

The above temporal delays are relevant to situations involving more complex movements. For example, if in a tracking situation the subject is required to keep a hand lever aligned with a dot on a screen, with the dot moving unpredictably, we typically see that the subject responds about 0.30 sec (approximately one RT) behind the movements of the dot; when the dot has been stationary and then suddenly (unpredictably) moves to the right, the subject remains stationary for one RT before he begins to follow the dot. In other situations, when the dot moves suddenly to the right for about 0.20 sec, and then suddenly reverses its direction to move back to the left, we see that the subject waits one RT before beginning his movement to the right and then *continues to move* for 0.20 sec before he can respond to the target's reversed direction. These findings suggest that whenever some event occurs unpredictably in the environment, the delay in initiating a response is about one RT, about 0.20–0.30 sec. This appears to be true for all of the sense modalities, but Chernikoff and Taylor (1952) have found that the RT to kinesthetic information was about 0.11 sec, somewhat faster than for visual and auditory information.

Time Required to Process Visual Information

In order to determine the time required to make use of visual feedback in the ongoing control of movement, Keele and Posner (1968) used a task in which subjects had to move a stylus from one small, circular target to another with vision. Subjects learned to do this task in either 0.15, 0.25, 0.35, or 0.45 sec. When the movements were well practiced, Keele and Posner would occasionally turn off the lights at the moment the subject left the starting position; they compared errors in hitting the target under conditions with and without vision. When the movement time was 0.15 sec, subjects missed the target *no more often* with the lights off than with the lights on; for the 0.25-sec movement, there was a slight advantage with the lights on, with the advantage of vision increasing as movement times increased further. Because withholding vision in the 0.15-sec movement did not affect errors, subjects apparently *could not use vision* to control movements this rapid even when vision was present. However, with the 0.25-sec movement, vision was effective in reducing errors. On this basis, the time required to make corrections in response to visual feedback is apparently between 0.15 and 0.25 sec, a range that agrees well with typical values for visual RT.

Time Required to Amend Movements

Slater-Hammel (1960) studied the time required to stop a preplanned movement. He had each subject hold his finger on a reaction key while he watched a clock whose hand made one revolution per sec. The clock started at 0, and the subject's job was to lift his finger off the key at the exact moment the clock hand reached 800 msec (0.80 sec). Occasionally, however, the clock hand would stop before reaching 800 msec; if it did, the subject was to inhibit his response and do nothing. Stopping the clock closer and closer to 800 msec rendered subjects less able to inhibit their responses. When the clock suddenly stopped 160 msec before the 800-msec mark (i.e., at 640 msec), subjects could inhibit their finger movement only half the time on the average. These data suggest that subjects "ordered" the finger response 160 msec (about one RT) before the finger movement; when the clock hand stopped after the movement had been ordered, the preplanned movement occurred without interruption.

Henry and Harrison (1961) make a similar point. Each subject made a rapid, horizontal, forward arm swing to trip a string in front of his shoulder. After the signal to begin the movement, a signal to stop the movement was given on some trials, with this stimulus coming on from 0.10 to 0.40 sec after the start signal. Subjects were unable to stop their movements unless the "stop" stimulus came on *before* the beginning of the movement, that is, during the RT for the movement. If the stimulus came on after this, the movement was performed without alteration.

These three studies make a number of very important points for the understanding of motor skills. First, it takes about one RT for an individual to be able to do anything about information that is presented while he is making a movement, whether that information be the vision of his own hand or the onset of a light. Second, if information provided by visual, auditory, or kinesthetic feedback indicates that he should change his response—either by stopping it altogether or by performing slight corrections—it requires about one RT for him to *begin* to initiate the changes. Taken together, these findings suggest that the first 0.20 or 0.30 sec of *any* movement must be "preprogrammed." This means that any information from the environment that indicates that the performer should change the response from that *originally intended* cannot be responded to until the movement has been under way for 0.3 to 0.5 sec.

ELIMINATING FEEDBACK
DELAYS: ANTICIPATION

In situations where a suddenly presented, unanticipated stimulus—either to initiate a movement or to change it—is delivered, it should be clear that individuals show rather severe delays in responding to it because of RT and psychological refractoriness. However, many of the situations present in skills involve situations in which the stimuli are *expected* or *anticipated*. A baseball is not presented suddenly to a batter, but rather is viewed for about 0.60 sec before its arrival at the plate. Through anticipation, the individual can ready himself for the upcoming stimuli and get his response under way in advance, thereby avoiding the drastic delays discussed above. A number of different types of anticipation have been outlined by Poulton (1957), and they are described below.

Types of Anticipation

Effector anticipation. In a task such as hitting a baseball, the batter must be able to anticipate how long the movement of the bat will take in order that the bat meet the ball over the plate, and the knowledge about the individual's own movement time is termed effector anticipation. Clearly, in order for the batter to know when to "give the motor command" to swing the bat, he must know how long that swing will take so that he can issue the command in advance at the appropriate time.

Receptor anticipation. Receptor anticipation involves the monitoring of relevant upcoming stimuli with the various receptors (e.g., eyes, ears). In hitting a baseball, the batter must watch the ball as it comes toward him, and he uses this *preview* as a basis for determining the time of initiation of his swing. If the batter did not have the ability to anticipate, he would respond to the arrival of the ball one RT late. Receptor anticipation is clearly important in skillful performances involving preview.

Perceptual anticipation. Perceptual anticipation occurs when there is some regularity in the upcoming events, but the individual does not have direct receptor information of these events. A good example is the drummer who must make a drum beat exactly 0.50 sec after the previous drum beat, without any direct sensory information concerning the passage of time. In these situations the regularity of the signals must be learned, and once learned, the performer does not need the direct vision of the upcoming events in order to anticipate them. The quarterback attempts to prevent the defensive team from perceptually anticipating the snap of the ball by varying the signal count; otherwise the defensive team could respond without making RT delays and speed up their performance greatly.

Anticipating in Skills

The skillful performer learns to anticipate in his performances whenever he can, the chief reason being that he must try to eliminate or reduce the drastic RT and refractoriness delays present when he does not anticipate. By anticipating in the ways described above, he can reduce the amount of attention required for the task, his performances become smoother and less labored, and he is more accurate in situations requiring timing. In fact, a skillful performer in many sports strives to prevent *his opponent* from anticipating by concealing the type of shot or pitch until the last moment, by hitting or pitching a ball with spin so that it behaves unpredictably, or by using unpredictable strategies. Thus anticipation is invaluable for skillful performance, largely because of the severe RT and refractoriness delays; being able to prevent anticipation in one's opponent gives a strong advantage.

AN EXAMPLE: PROCESSING
FEEDBACK IN BATTING

How does the evidence concerning various feedback processing delays and anticipation relate to understanding how individuals perform complex motor skills? Consider hitting a baseball. It has been shown that the time from the beginning of the bat movement until the bat crosses the plate is about 0.10 sec in good hitters. Also, we know that the decision as to whether to swing or not to swing, including all of the decisions about the height and velocity of the swing, must be made before one RT

(0.20 sec) before the movement starts. This means that the batter must decide all of the details of the swing 0.30 sec before the ball reaches the plate (0.10 sec for movement time and 0.20 sec for RT). Also, the time from when the ball leaves the pitcher's hand until it crosses the plate is about 0.60 sec for good pitchers. If the decisions about the swing must be made at least 0.30 sec before ball contact, the final decision must be made by the time the ball has traveled half way to the plate. Any changes after this point in the ball's position that were not accounted for in the decision (such as a sudden lateral movement, as with the "knuckle ball") cannot be responded to.

Those close to baseball may have noticed that portions of the swing actually start long before the point indicated in Fig. 10.3, perhaps even as the pitcher is in the act of his throw. However, these preliminary movements are performed to make the swing forceful and are performed *whether or not* the batter actually decides to complete the swing at the ball; thus the stride and hip movement are not considered part of the programmed act of the swing. However, as the ball approaches, the batter must eventually make his decision on the basis of the ball's location and velocity as to whether to swing (i.e., to "break" his wrists), and this final decision must be made 0.30 sec before the ball comes over the plate.

What should be the effect of a fast versus a slow swing on hitting, assuming that the two swings begin at the same place? Some would argue that the "home-run" swing should be less accurate, but the theory actually predicts the opposite. If the movement time for the swing is reduced from 0.10 sec to, say,

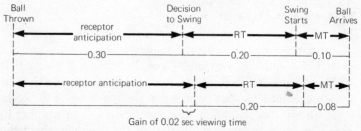

Gain of 0.02 sec viewing time

Fig. 10.3 Hypothetical example of the temporal sequencing of events in hitting a baseball.

0.08 sec by speeding it up, the batter should be able to delay his decision about the nature of the swing by 0.02 sec as shown in the bottom of Fig. 10.3. Therefore, the faster swing should result in an additional 0.02 sec (approximately 2 ft of ball travel) to view the ball and to make decisions about its flight, which should lead to increased accuracy in hitting the ball. Schmidt (1969) varied the movement speed of a hitting response in a laboratory task and found that increased movement speed resulted in greater accuracy in meeting the target at the correct time, which is consistent with the ideas presented above.

THE MOTOR PROGRAM

We demonstrated earlier that delays in processing information prevented the performer from making changes in the originally-intended movement until approximately 0.3 to 0.5 sec had elapsed.[1] Since this environmental information cannot, therefore, be the basis for the control of the movement, motor behaviorists have invoked the notion of the *motor program* as the mechanism that produces these movements. The motor program is thought to be a set of stored muscle commands that, when activated, determine the muscle commands that determine the movement. Actually, the evidence about the delays in processing information do not "prove" the existence of the motor program, since to do so one would have to show that (1) either there is no environmental feedback and the movement can be carried out or that (2) such feedback is present but is not used. Strictly speaking, neither condition has been shown for human performance.

On the other hand, perhaps the strongest human evidence for the motor program comes from the simple finding that an

[1] The subject can commit an error in two ways: (1) ordering the wrong motor program, and (2) ordering the correct motor program, but executing it improperly. The statement that the movement cannot be corrected by feedback until 0.30 sec has elapsed applies to the first type of error. There is mounting evidence that the second type of error can be corrected to some extent, using feedback, via the muscle-spindle system; unfortunately, a discussion of these processes is beyond the scope of this book.

individual can initiate, carry out, and stop a movement to a target all within a movement time of less than 0.10 sec, which is clearly less than one RT. In these movements how does the individual know when to "issue" the command to stop the limb? One hypothesis is that he moves his hand along until feedback from vision and kinesthesis tells the subject that he is at such a location that stop instructions should be sent. Since the time for such processes is about one RT, reliance on visual or kinesthetic stimuli would cause the movement to begin to stop *well after* the desired end point. Therefore, the instructions to stop the movement had to be issued before the movement's beginning. The motor program is assumed to contain these instructions to start, carry out, and stop the movement. When the command to perform the movement is issued from the "executive," the program is carried out, giving the commands to the correct muscles in the proper order and at the proper time so that the movement is as desired. Environmental feedback information, including information that the wrong movement has been chosen or that the response should be inhibited, cannot be processed and the movement goes on as programmed.

Nonhuman Evidence

In spite of the evidence that individuals can initiate and terminate a movement that is less than one RT in length, motor behaviorists have demanded more evidence of the motor program, and some have looked at other species for such data. Wilson (1961) cut all of the afferent (i.e., feedback) nerves from a locust's wings, related muscles, and joints so that the insect received no information about the movements of his own wings. Electrical stimulation of a cluster of nerve cells near the head initiated a rhythmic, sustained oscillation of the wings resembling flying. With the feedback channels cut, the movement must have been produced by the stored commands, direct evidence that motor programs exist in insects.

Although the insect data suggest strongly that motor programs do exist, these conclusions seem to be limited to programs that can probably be considered "innate." However, the notion of the motor program for human beings seems to be more complex, involving actions that are clearly learned. For example, we speak of the motor program for kicking a football or throwing a baseball as being a set of commands structured as a result of learning and stored for future use. However, there are no nonhuman data that provide evidence for acquired motor programs; such findings would add considerably to the body of knowledge concerning motor control.

Characteristics of the Motor Program

Duration. We assume from the temporal limitations in processing feedback that the *minimum* time the motor program can be in force is about one RT. That is, when the movement begins, events during the movement that might require the individual to modify his originally intended program can begin to have an effect only after one RT, or about 0.20 sec; however, this estimate is probably too low for most of the responses in motor skills because events to which a change in program is required may not occur until the movement has been under way for some time. Therefore, the minimum time a program would be operating is one RT plus the time the program was under way before any signal to change it. For example, a movement that normally takes 0.60 sec might be under way for about 0.30 sec before the individual detects that he has ordered the wrong movement and that it is going to be incorrect, in which case he could just begin to change the program in 0.30 plus 0.20 sec (RT), and the program would be in force for 0.50 sec. When one considers that most of the hitting and kicking responses in sports are very much quicker than 0.50 sec in duration, motor programs would appear to have an important role in skills.

What is the *maximum* time that a program could be in force? Correcting movements in progress probably requires that the individual *attend* to the stimuli that are to signal the change. In many tasks, the performer decreases the amount of attention he pays to the task as practice progresses (automatization, Chapter 4), and therefore, with limited attention to the task, the program could control the response for much longer than the 0.50 sec mentioned above, perhaps for a few sec or more. If the movement becomes wildly incorrect (such as in walking movements when the individual trips on a curb), feedback could be used to modify the movements. Therefore, there seems to be no theoretical upper limit on the duration of a motor program, and one of the beneficial aspects of practice is that the performer develops "good" motor programs that can carry out long strings of movement in the absence of attention, allowing him to attend to other aspects of the environment (e.g., to talk to a friend while walking).

Effect of movement variables.   The motor program notion has predictions for a number of movement variables. For example, any variable that causes the movement time to increase will increase the time available to use feedback to correct movements while they are in progress. Schmidt (1969) has shown that increasing the movement distance, decreasing the movement speed, and increasing the load on the movement (all of which increase movement time) decreased the subject's reliance on the motor program. Also, Schmidt and Russell (1972) found that two movements with the same movement *time*, but with different movement *distances* (the longer distance producing a movement of greater *speed*), utilized the program to the same degree. These data suggest that the use of a motor program is determined primarily by the *time* over which the individual moves and that the quality and type of movement has little to do with the use of feedback to modify the originally intended response.

Learning and the Motor Program

A major question concerning the motor program is how its role changes over practice at a given task. One possibility is that the role of the program increases, in that longer and longer segments of behavior are programmed (i.e., performed without intervention from feedback), with the primary advantage being that it frees attention to perform other tasks. However, a second possibility is that the individual programs less as practice continues because he has learned to use feedback more effectively and can make within-movement corrections in later practice that he could not in earlier practice. Thus, learning that certain patterns of feedback indicate that an error was occurring, with the subsequent and rapid correction of it, could allow the individual to program less as a function of practice.

Pew (1966), in an experiment described in Chapter 4, had subjects attempt to keep a dot in the center of a screen by the appropriate pressing of two buttons, the right button making the dot accelerate to the right and the left button making it accelerate to the left. In early practice, subjects were operating in a closed-loop mode, in which they made a single response, waited for its feedback consequences, made another single response, and so on, so that the movements were quite jerky and performance was poor. However, in later practice, subjects had shifted to an open-loop (programming) mode, in which they made a series of rapid alternate button presses, each of which could not have been produced in response to visual feedback because it was far too fast (about 8 per sec). Since the movements were being performed too rapidly for each button press to be produced in response to visual stimuli, the subjects had developed a string of actions that was governed by the motor program, which was not dependent, for at least short periods of time, on feedback stimuli. Thus, Pew's evidence suggests that the learner develops more efficient motor programs as a function of practice and that he uses feedback less frequently than he did in early practice. Recent data from Schmidt and McCabe (1974), using the index of preprogramming (IP) (Schmidt, 1972c) as a measure of the amount of feedback involvement in movement, supported the same conclusion in a discrete task.

REFERENCES

Adams, J. A. 1961. The second facet of forgetting: A review of warm-up decrement. *Psychological Bulletin* 58, 257–273.

_____. 1967. *Human Memory*. New York: McGraw-Hill.

_____. 1971. A closed-loop theory of motor learning. *Journal of Motor Behavior* 3, 111–150.

_____, and Creamer, L. R. 1962. Anticipatory timing of continuous and discrete responses. *Journal of Experimental Psychology* 63, 84–90.

_____, and Dijkstra, S. 1966. Short-term memory for motor responses. *Journal of Experimental Psychology* 71, 314–318.

_____, and Hufford, L. E. 1962. Contributions of a part-task trainer to the learning and relearning of a time-shared flight maneuver. *Human Factors* 4, 159–170.

_____, and Reynolds, B. 1954. Effect of shift in distribution of practice conditions following interpolated rest. *Journal of Experimental Psychology* 47, 32–36.

Alderman, R. B. 1965. Influence of local fatigue on speed and accuracy in motor learning. *Research Quarterly* 36, 131–140.

Ammons, R. B. 1951. Effects of pre-practice activities on rotary pursuit performance. *Journal of Experimental Psychology* 41, 187–191.

Ascoli, K. M., and Schmidt, R. A. 1969. Proactive interference in short-term motor retention. *Journal of Motor Behavior* 1, 29–36.

Atkinson, R. C., and Shiffrin, R. M. 1971. The control of short-term memory. *Scientific American* 225, 82–90.

Bachman, J. C. 1961. Specificity vs. generality in learning and performing two large muscle motor tasks. *Research Quarterly* 32, 3–11.

Bahrick, H. P.; Fitts, P. M.; and Briggs, G. E. 1957. Learning curves—facts or artifacts. *Psychological Bulletin* 54, 256–268.

Bahrick, H. P., and Shelley, C. H. 1954. Time-sharing as an index of automatization. *Journal of Experimental Psychology* 56, 288–293.

Barnett, M. L.; Ross, D.; Schmidt, R. A.; and Todd, B. 1973. Motor skills learning and the specificity of training principle. *Research Quarterly* 44, 440–447.

Bilodeau, E. A., and Bilodeau, I. McD. 1958a. Variable frequency of knowledge of results and the learning of simple skill. *Journal of Experimental Psychology* 55, 379–385.

_____. 1958b. Variation of temporal intervals among critical events in five studies of knowledge of results. *Journal of Experimental Psychology* 55, 603–612.

_____, and Schumsky, D. A. 1959. Some effects of introducing and withdrawing knowledge of results early and late in practice. *Journal of Experimental Psychology* 58, 142–144.

Bilodeau, E. A., and Rosenbach, J. H. 1953. Acquisition of response proficiency as a function of rounding error in information feedback. *USAF Human Resources Research Center Research Bulletin*, no. 53-21.

Bilodeau, I. McD. 1956. Accuracy of a simple positioning response with variation in the number of trials by which knowledge of results is delayed. *American Journal of Psychology* 69, 434–437.

_____. 1969. Information feedback. In E. A. Bilodeau, ed., *Principles of Skill Acquisition*. New York: Academic.

Blankenship, W. C. 1952. *Transfer effects in neuro-muscular responses involving choice*. M.A. dissertation, University of California.

Boulter, L. R. 1964. Evaluation of mechanisms in delay of knowledge of results. *Canadian Journal of Psychology* 18, 281–291.

Bourne, L. E., and Bunderson, C. V. 1963. Effects of delay of informative feedback and length of postfeedback interval on concept identification. *Journal of Experimental Psychology* 65, 1–5.

Briggs, G. E. 1957. Retroactive inhibition as a function of the degree of original and interpolated learning. *Journal of Experimental Psychology* 53, 60–67.

_____, and Brogden, W. S. 1954. The effect of component practice on performance in a lever-positioning skill. *Journal of Experimental Psychology* 48, 375–380.

Briggs, G. E., and Waters, L. K. 1958. Training and transfer as a function of component interaction. *Journal of Experimental Psychology* 56, 492–500.

Broer, M. 1958. Effectiveness of a general basic skills curriculum for junior high school girls. *Research Quarterly* 29, 379–388.

Brown, J. 1958. Some tests of the decay theory of immediate memory. *Quarterly Journal of Experimental Psychology* 10, 12–21.

Bryan, W. L., and Harter, N. 1899. Studies on the telegraphic language. The acquisition of a hierarchy of habits. *Psychological Review* 6, 345–375.

Caplan, C. S. 1970. *The influence of physical fatigue on massed versus distributed motor learning.* Paper presented at the American Association for Health, Physical Education, and Recreation National Conference, Seattle.

Carron, A. V. 1967. Performance and learning in a discrete motor task under massed versus distributed practice. Ph.D. dissertation, University of California.

Chernikoff, R., and Taylor, F. V. 1952. Reaction time to kinesthetic stimulation resulting from sudden arm displacement. *Journal of Experimental Psychology* 43, 1–8.

Crossman, E. R. F. W. 1959. A theory of the acquisition of speed-skill. *Ergonomics* 2, 153–166.

Davies, D. R. 1945. The effect of tuition upon the process of learning a complex motor skill. *Journal of Educational Psychology* 36, 352–365.

Deese, J. 1967. *General Psychology.* Boston: Allyn & Bacon.

Duncan, C. P., and Underwood, B. J. 1953. Retention of transfer in motor learning after 24 hours and after 14 months. *Journal of Experimental Psychology* 46, 445–452.

Ellis, M. J. 1972. *Why People Play.* Englewood Cliffs, N.J.: Prentice-Hall.

Ells, J. G. 1969. *Attentional requirements of movement control.* Ph.D. dissertation, University of Oregon.

Espenschade, A. 1940. Motor performance in adolescence. *Social Research in Child Development Monographs* 5, 1–33.

Fitts, P. M. 1964. Perceptual-motor skill learning. In A. W. Melton, ed., *Categories of Human Learning.* New York: Academic.

————, **and Posner, M. I.** 1967. *Human Performance.* Belmont, Calif.: Brooks-Cole.

Fleishman, E. A. 1965. The description and prediction of perceptual-motor skill learning. In R. Glaser, ed., *Training Research and Education.* New York: Wiley.

————, **and Hempel, W. E., Jr.** 1954. Changes in factor structure of a complex psychomotor test as a function of practice. *Psychometrika* 18, 239–252.

————, **and Parker, S. F.** 1962. Factors in the retention and relearning of perceptual-motor skill. *Journal of Experimental Psychology* 64, 215–276.

————, and **Rich, S.** 1963. Role of kinesthetic and spacial-visual abilities in perceptual motor learning. *Journal of Experimental Psychology* 66, 6–11.

Forscher, B. K. 1963. Chaos in the brickyard. *Science* 142, 3590.

Godwin, M. A., and Schmidt, R. A. 1971. Muscular fatigue and discrete motor learning. *Research Quarterly* 42, 374–383.

Gross, E. A.; Griesel, D. C.; and Stull, G. A. 1956. Relationship between two motor educability tests, a strength test, and wrestling ability after eight weeks' instruction. *Research Quarterly* 27, 395–402.

Hellyer, S. 1962. Supplementary report: Frequency of stimulus presentation and short-term decrement in recall. *Journal of Experimental Psychology* 64, 650.

Henry, F. M. 1961. Reaction time-movement time correlations. *Perceptual and Motor Skills* 12, 63–66.

————. 1968. Specificity vs. generality in learning motor skill. In R. C. Brown and G. S. Kenyon, eds., *Classical Studies on Physical Activity*. Englewood Cliffs, N.J.: Prentice-Hall.

————, and **Harrison, J. S.** 1961. Refractoriness of a fast movement. *Perceptual and Motor Skills* 13, 351–354.

Hull, C. L. 1943. *Principles of Psychology*. New York: Appleton.

Irion, A. L. 1948. The relation of "set" to retention. *Psychological Review* 55, 336–341.

————. 1966. A brief history of research on the acquisition of skill. In E. A. Bilodeau, ed., *Acquisition of Skill*. New York: Academic, chap. 1.

James, W. 1890. *The Principles of Psychology*. New York: Holt, vol. 1.

Keele, S. W., and Posner, M. I. 1968. Processing feedback in rapid movements. *Journal of Experimental Psychology* 77, 353–363.

Keppel, G., and Underwood, B. J. 1962. Proactive inhibition in short-term retention of single items. *Journal of Verbal Learning and Verbal Behavior* 1, 153–161.

Kimble, G. A. 1949. Performance and reminiscence in motor learning as a function of the degree of distribution of practice. *Journal of Experimental Psychology* 39, 500–510.

Lachman, R. 1960. The model in theory construction. *Psychological Review* 67, 113–129.

Lersten, K. C. 1968. Transfer of movement components in a motor learning task. *Research Quarterly* 39, 575–581.

————. 1969. Retention of skill on the Rho apparatus after one year. *Research Quarterly* 40, 418–419.

Lewis, D.; McAllister, D. E.; and Adams, J. A. 1951. Facilitation and interference in performance on the modified Mashburn apparatus: I, After-effects of varying the amount of original learning. *Journal of Experimental Psychology* 41, 247–260.

Lindeburg, F. A. 1949. A study of the degree of transfer between quickening exercises and other movements. *Research Quarterly* 20, 180–189.

Locke, E. A.; Cartledge, N.; and Koeppel, J. 1968. Motivational effects of knowledge of results: A goal-setting phenomenon? *Psychological Bulletin* 70, 474–485.

Lordahl, D. S., and Archer, J. E. 1958. Transfer effects on a rotary pursuit task as a function of first task difficulty. *Journal of Experimental Psychology* 56, 421–426.

Lotter, W. S. 1960. Interrelationships among reaction times and speeds of movement in different limbs. *Research Quarterly* 31, 147–155.

McAllister, D. E. 1952. Retroactive facilitation and interference as a function of the level of learning. *American Journal of Psychology* 65, 218–232.

McCloy, C. H. 1934. The measurement of general motor capacity and general motor ability. *Research Quarterly Supplement* 5, 46–61.

Martin, H. A. 1970. Long-term retention of a discrete motor task. M.A. dissertation, University of Maryland.

Meyers, J. 1967. Retention of balance coordination learning as influenced by extended lay-offs. *Research Quarterly* 38, 72–78.

Mohr, D. R., and Barrett, M. E. 1962. Effect of knowledge of mechanical principles in learning to perform intermediate swimming skills. *Research Quarterly* 33, 574–580.

Nacson, J., and Schmidt, R. A. 1971. The activity-set hypothesis for warm-up decrement. *Journal of Motor Behavior* 3, 1–16.

Namikas, G., and Archer, J. E. 1960. Motor skill transfer as a function of intertask interval and pretransfer task difficulty. *Journal of Experimental Psychology* 59, 109–112.

Neisser, U. 1967. *Cognitive Psychology*. New York: Appleton.

Peterson, L. R., and Peterson, M. J. 1959. Short-term retention of individual verbal items. *Journal of Experimental Psychology* 58, 193–198.

Pew, R. W. 1966. Acquisition of hierarchical control over the temporal organization of a skill. *Journal of Experimental Psychology* 71, 764–771.

Platt, J. R. 1964. Strong inference. *Science* 146, 347–353.

Polya, G. 1954. *Mathematics and Plausible Reasoning*. Princeton, N.J.: Princeton University Press, p. 10.

Poulton, E. C. 1957. On-prediction in skilled movements. *Psychological Bulletin* 54, 467–478.

Richardson, A. 1967. Mental practice: A review and discussion. *Research Quarterly* 38, 95–107.

Ryan, E. D. 1962. Retention of stabilometer and pursuit rotor skills. *Research Quarterly* 33, 46–51.

Salmoni, A. G. 1973. Attention demands of a linear motor response. Unpublished research, Motor Behavior Laboratory, University of Michigan.

Schmidt, R. A. 1966. Transfer of motor learning. Unpublished paper, University of Illinois.

————. 1968. Proactive inhibition in retention of discrete motor skill. Proceedings of the International Society of Sports Psychology, Washington, D.C., October.

————. 1969. Movement time as a determiner of timing accuracy. *Journal of Experimental Psychology* 79, 43–47.

————. 1971. Retroactive interference and amount of original learning in verbal and motor tasks. *Research Quarterly* 42, 314–326.

————. 1972a. Experimental psychology. In R. N. Singer, ed., *The Psychomotor Domain: Movement Behavior*. Philadelphia: Lea & Febiger.

————. 1972b. The case against learning and forgetting scores. *Journal of Motor Behavior* 4, 79–88.

————. 1972c. The index of preprogramming (IP): A statistical method for evaluating the role of feedback in simple movements. *Psychonomic Science* 27, 83–85.

————, and Ascoli, K. M. 1970. Intertrial intervals and motor short-term memory. *Research Quarterly* 41, 432–438.

————, and McCabe, J. F. 1974. Changes in motor program utilization over extended practice. Unpublished research. Motor Behavior Laboratory, University of Michigan.

————, and Nacson, J. 1971. Further tests of the activity-set hypothesis, for warm-up decrement. *Journal of Experimental Psychology* 90, 56–64.

————, and Russell, D. G. 1972. Movement velocity and movement time as determiners of the degree of preprogramming in simple movements. *Journal of Experimental Psychology* 96, 315–320.

————, and White, J. L. 1972. Evidence for an error detection mechanism in motor skills: A test of Adams' closed-loop theory. *Journal of Motor Behavior* 4, 143–153.

————, and Wrisberg, C. A. 1971. The activity-set hypothesis for warm-up decrement in a movement speed task. *Journal of Motor Behavior* 3, 318–325.

————. 1973. Further tests of the Adams' closed-loop theory: Response-produced feedback and the error detection mechanism. *Journal of Motor Behavior* 5, 155–164.

Schutz, R. W., and Roy, E. A. 1973. Absolute error: The devil in disguise. *Journal of Motor Behavior* 5, 141–153.

Seymour, W. D. 1954. Experiments on the acquisition of industrial skills. *Occupational Psychology* 28, 77–89.

Singer, R. N. 1968. *Motor Learning and Human Performance*. New York: Macmillan.

————. 1972. *Readings in Motor Learning*. Philadelphia: Lea & Febiger.

Skinner, B. F. 1956. A case history in scientific method. *American Psychologist* 11, 221–233.

Slater-Hammel, A. T. 1960. Reliability, accuracy and refractoriness of a transit reaction. *Research Quarterly* 31, 217–228.

Snoddy, G. S. 1926. Learning and stability. *Journal of Applied Psychology* 10, 1–36.

Stelmach, G. E. 1969a. Efficiency of motor learning as a function of intertrial rest. *Research Quarterly* 40, 198–202.

————. 1969b. Prior positioning responses as a factor in short-term retention of a simple motor task. *Journal of Experimental Psychology* 81, 523–526.

————, and Walsh, M. F. 1972. Response biasing as a function of duration and extent of positioning acts. *Journal of Experimental Psychology* 92, 354–359.

Szafran, J., and Welford, A. T. 1950. On the relation between transfer and difficulty of initial task. *Quarterly Journal of Experimental Psychology* 2, 88–96.

Taub, E., and Berman, A. J. 1968. Movement and learning in the absence of sensory feedback. In S. J. Freedman, ed., *The Neuropsychology of Spatially Oriented Behavior*. Homewood, Ill.: Dorsey.

Trowbridge, M. H., and Cason, H. 1932. An experimental study of Thorndike's theory of learning. *Journal of General Psychology* 7, 245–260.

Trumbo, D.; Ulrich, L.; and Noble, M. E. 1965. Verbal coding and display coding in the acquisition and retention of tracking skill. *Journal of Applied Psychology* 49, 368–375.

Underwood, B. J. 1957. Interference and forgetting. *Psychological Review* 64, 49–60.

Weinberg, D. R.; Guy, D. E.; and Tupper, R. W. 1964. Variation of postfeedback interval in simple motor learning. *Journal of Experimental Psychology* 67, 98–99.

Welford, A. T. 1968. *Fundamentals of Skill*. London: Methuen.

Whitley, J. D. 1970. Effects of practice distribution on learning a fine motor task. *Research Quarterly* 41, 576–583.

Wilson, D. M. 1961. The central nervous control of flight in a locust. *Journal of Experimental Biology* 38, 471–490.

Woodward, P. 1943. An experimental study of transfer of training in motor learning. *Journal of Applied Psychology* 27, 12–20.

Woodworth, R. S. 1899. The accuracy of voluntary movement. *Psychological Monographs* 3 (whole no. 13).

INDEX